Praise for *Invincible*

"A treasure of empowering insight and wisdom! In *Invincible*, Howard Falco has written a guidebook for the optimal state of mind. If you are looking to take command and change your experience in a positive way, this book will help reinvigorate your mind and inspire happiness, creativity, and a new belief in what is possible for you and your life. It's a must-read!"

—Jon Gordon, 17-time bestselling author of *The One Truth*

"Sometimes a book comes along that changes everything . . . *Invincible* is one of those books! Howard consistently empowers and enlightens. *Invincible* is a true masterpiece, filled with practical wisdom and clear-cut strategies for creating a life of calm confidence, inner compassion, and clarity of vision. Howard's insights—when applied—will awaken your dormant greatness for you to achieve inevitable success."

—Dr. Darren Weissman, developer of The LifeLine Technique® and author of *The Power of Infinite Love and Gratitude*

"Howard Falco is a rare and gifted spiritual teacher. *Invincible* is a literal playbook for anyone seeking a deeper, more meaningful experience of life. His book is clearly laid out and highly accessible to anyone on the path toward living and creating their life more consciously. *Invincible* moves you beyond the false notion that you are nothing more than the sum of your past and your heredity, to give you the power and simple and direct steps to master your mind and your best life."

—Jackie Woodside, spiritual teacher, TEDx speaker, and author of *Calming the Chaos*

"*Invincible* is more than a book; it's a blueprint for success for those who know they're meant to play a bigger, bolder game but haven't yet closed the gap. In the book, you'll find principles, secrets, and, most importantly, a step-by-step framework from one of the best teachers on the planet who walks the walk of his work every day and teaches you how to do the same. Warning: your life might significantly change in the most positive and best of ways!"

—Tommy Baker, coach and author of *The 1% Rule*

"Howard Falco has done it again! *Invincible* shows you how to use your mind, your most powerful tool, to perform to your potential. This book will help you develop the invincible mindset necessary to achieve your goals in sports, business, and life."

—Jeff Janssen, author of *The Team Captain's Leadership Manual* and president of the Janssen Sports Leadership Center

"*Invincible* is a powerful book on possibility! I know firsthand. After working with Howard on mental strength, I became a champion on the LPGA Tour. If you are looking for game-changing insights on mindset and personal power, this book is it!"

—Mel Reid, LPGA Tour professional and champion, and NBC Sports analyst

"*Invincible* is a blueprint to achieving excellence. This book will help athletes of all skill levels improve their mindset and mental strength."

—Steve Dahlby, top-ranked PGA teaching professional and swing coach on the PGA Tour

"As a former professional athlete, I understand the significant impact the mind has on attaining next-level success. Howard's thoughts and work on the power of mindset, when it comes to sports and life, are second to none. His new book *Invincible* is a priceless guide for anyone seeking to be in the highest state of mind possible for whatever they are looking to accomplish. I'm proud to say that I've worked with Howard, and only wish I had had the opportunity to experience his teachings and this mentality while I was still playing!"

—Rich Aurilia, former Major League Baseball player and All-Star for the San Francisco Giants, and NBC Sports commentator

"In the realm of personal development, Howard Falco's new book *Invincible* stands out as a game changer! Having studied personal development for over thirty years, and having worked with leaders like Jack Canfield, Tony Robbins, Brian Tracy, and Brendan Burchard, I can confidently say Howard's teachings are on another level with the information in this book. His insights have been invaluable in helping me, as a business owner, see the connection between my results and my state of mind and beliefs! Howard's work is essential for anyone striving to not just achieve success, but to actually feel it and embody it."

—Michael Maske, president and CEO of ZM Medical

"Working with Howard on mental strength was a game changer during my MLB career. In *Invincible*, he shares many of the secrets he taught me about achieving the best state of mind for optimal performance. The great thing is that these strategies work for any walk of life and any situation in life. This book is a POWERFUL and LIFE-CHANGING read!"

—Brandon Guyer, former Major League Baseball player for
the Cleveland Guardians, and peak performance and mindset coach

"My work with Howard had a great impact on my mindset and led to great results in my career, including a breakthrough win at AT&T Pebble Beach Pro-Am in 2020. This book is sure to help anyone looking to reach their true potential!"

—Nick Taylor, professional golfer and four-time winner on the PGA Tour

"Howard's work on mindfulness holds the power to change your mind and your results in the best of ways."

—Allen Lazard, NFL wide receiver for the New York Jets

"After a near-fatal car crash that took my left arm, Howard's work single-handedly changed my outlook and my life. In *Invincible*, he has put together a brilliant, logical, step-by-step guide to create the highest version of YOU! Regardless of your past, what happened, or where you came from, this work has the ability to catapult you into the true unlimited person that you're destined to be that, prior to this wisdom, you may have not known existed. An incredible, life-changing resource!"

—Michael Fine, acclaimed international Hatha yoga instructor
and motivational speaker

Also by Howard Falco

I AM: The Power of Discovering Who You Really Are

Time in a Bottle: Mastering the Experience of Life

INVINCIBLE

The Mindset of

Infinite Potential

and the Secret

to Inevitable Success

HOWARD FALCO

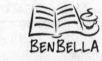

BenBella Books, Inc.
Dallas, TX

BENBELLA

BenBella Books, Inc.
8080 N. Central Expressway
Suite 1700
Dallas, TX 75206
benbellabooks.com
Send feedback to feedback@benbellabooks.com

BenBella is a federally registered trademark.

Printed in the United States of America
10 9 8 7 6 5 4 3 2 1

Library of Congress Control Number: 2024039025
ISBN 9781637746073 (trade paperback)
ISBN 9781637746080 (electronic)

Editing by Victoria Carmody
Copyediting by Jennifer Greenstein
Proofreading by Jenny Bridges and Marissa Wold Uhrina
Text design and composition by Jordan Koluch
Cover design by Morgan Carr
Printed by Lake Book Manufacturing

**Special discounts for bulk sales are available.
Please contact bulkorders@benbellabooks.com.**

This book and the love that flows through it
are a beautiful testament to my mother,
Maureen Sue Buley, who passed on April 12, 2023.

Her unconditional love and endless wisdom
made me who I AM.

I am eternally grateful for her.

If you knew how powerful you really are, you would never stop smiling.

To humanity: Exalt thyself.

Contents

PART TWO: BREAKTHROUGH

PART THREE: NEXT-LEVEL MINDFULNESS

INTRODUCTION

Welcome to the Invincible State of Mind

> The self-confidence of the warrior is not the
> self-confidence of the ordinary man. The av-
> erage man seeks certainty in the eyes of the
> onlooker and calls that self-confidence. The
> warrior seeks impeccability in his own eyes
> and calls that humbleness. The average man
> is hooked to his fellow men, while the war-
> rior is hooked only to infinity.
>
> —Carlos Castaneda

What if you embraced a mindset that opened the door to unlimited possibilities for your life? What if you knew in every fiber of your being that this mindset could release you, enabling you to more freely create any experience or dream that you desire for yourself? What if you built so much confidence in this approach that you worried less about your future and instead used your time and energy to create and enjoy the life you really want? What if you came to understand so much about how life is working for you that you could master any challenge and stay confident about your ultimate success in the process? If you did these things, you would be the master of your mind. You would open the door to a new way of understanding yourself and the world.

This book is an invitation to the awareness that will help you enter the most optimal state of mind, energy, and action. The invincible mindset is a place where you know how to handle any circumstance with the peace and grace of a Zen master. At the same time, this is a state of understanding that reveals how to create your desires like any top creative person in the world. In the pages that follow, you will learn a sacred and peaceful way of being that will take you to a new level of perception, experience, creation, and results. A place of flow and intuition, where thought and intention merge seamlessly with creation. The state of self-mastery.

The way your experience of life will unfold for you from this moment forward is not just about who you were in the past. It is not about projecting who you'll be in the future. Your experience is predominantly determined in this moment by how you decide to see and believe in who you are *now*. You see, this untouched moment is your single greatest gift: a fresh canvas and the never-ending opportunity to define, declare, and demonstrate who you choose to be. This is expressed by the primordial thought "I AM" and what you believe is true about yourself from this moment forward.

YOU ARE ALWAYS CAPABLE OF MORE

Do you feel there is more inside you that is waiting to come out and be experienced? Do you want to create a more fulfilling and peaceful way of life? If the answer is yes to either of these questions, know that these words are here to help guide you in that effort. Life does listen. Anxiety, worry, pressure, or any concern about your past or your future can be overcome. Opening to a new perspective has the power to positively change your entire life.

You can conquer your doubts, worries, and fears.

You can achieve new results in your life and shift the probabilities of your future.

You can learn to master your mind.

THE IMPORTANCE OF SEEKING WISDOM

The knowledge that has brought you to this moment in your life may not get you to the future experiences you desire. There is always new information to learn. For real, positive change to take hold in your life, you must initiate it by profoundly shifting the way you think and act. To change your mindset and behavior, you must change the way you perceive your circumstances. You must change the way you see your world, and most importantly, you must change the way you see yourself. This shift in perspective is what I call "next-level mindfulness."

The intent of this book is to guide you through a step-by-step process of understanding that leads to this transformational shift in perception and awareness. The purpose is to bring you to the greatest state of clarity on how life works and, as a result of this clarity, to a higher state of mental empowerment. The material is here to help ensure that your mindset—your awareness, energy, and actions—aligns more harmoniously with exactly what you are looking to create.

The process of embracing this mindset involves a tremendous amount of will, courage, belief, and, most importantly, patience. However, when you combine your desire to experience more of your infinite potential with a new, enriched understanding of how life works, you will be able to summon endless willpower! When you realize what is possible for you, and how life is continually supporting you at every step of your journey, you will courageously meet, work through, and overcome even the most daunting challenges you encounter.

"Knowing yourself is the beginning of all wisdom."

—Aristotle

THE NEXT EVOLUTION OF MIND

Today, millions of people are seeking a more effective way to deal with the turmoil and negativity of the world and in turn live a more empowered life. They are looking for a new mental approach to handling the seemingly never-ending onslaught of public health issues, political division, global military conflicts, and general suffering in the world. They may be troubled by work, business or financial stress, athletic pressures, or relationship disharmony and may be searching for new ways to simply find peace and contentment. Many are searching for a better way to navigate major challenges, understand and rise above life's chaos, and achieve a sense of purpose and the experiences they imagine for themselves.

Surface-level quotes, platitudes, and motivational catch-phrases that float past you as you scroll through your social media feed may no longer be doing the job of truly inspiring you or providing the answers that move the needle on your desired results. The mind of one who truly seeks answers is looking for a richer, deeper knowledge about life that works in terms of a better state of mind. The goal of so many is to stay inspired and energized and find an understanding that creates hope and ignites the creative desires of the soul.

Having counseled and coached thousands of people over the last twenty years, I've seen and heard just about every life circumstance, tragedy, and challenge imaginable. I've worked with those dealing with relationship heartbreak and unspeakable grief and helped them overcome regret or insecurity and find love and peace again. I've worked with business executives and struggling entrepreneurs and helped them find success. And I've worked with some of the top professional athletes in the world, helping them shift their mindsets and break through to higher levels of performance so they could achieve championships on the world's biggest stages.

In each case, and with each person I've worked with, the process is the same. The secret of the mindset shift and ultimate path to success I teach them is rooted in a certain change in how they look at the world and who they are. It's about realizing how this shift in identity connects to *every energetic encounter on their road of life.* This awareness is the nucleus of your inner power! It is this vital expansion of mind and divine awareness that I am honored to be offering you in a step-by-step process throughout this book.

MY JOURNEY TO THIS STATE OF UNDERSTANDING

As a young child, I was always extremely curious about life. I was that kid in class who was always raising his hand and questioning, questioning, questioning. As I grew older, I voraciously sought the answers to life's biggest and deepest questions. In 1981, at the age of fourteen, I had what was my first spiritual experience. It was that moment that sparked the fire in me to learn and understand more about how life works.

INTRODUCTION

My aunt and uncle invited me to go with my cousin on a fishing trip to the beautiful Northwoods of Minnesota. Our destination was a very remote place called Bear Island Lake, in the northeastern part of the state, less than a hundred miles from the Canadian border. They had rented an old, weathered cabin that sat on the edge of the water. The land-scape could have been a scene from the opening of a great novel or movie. It was as far away as I had ever been from the suburbs and city lights of Chicago.

We drove up to the cabin at dusk, unloaded the car, and unpacked. Afterward, everyone was exhausted and ready for bed but me. I wanted to explore my new surroundings. So I went straight out, walked down to the long end of an old, creaky, wooden boat dock, and just stopped and stared out into the darkness of the massive lake before me.

The scene didn't seem real. It was my first experience with the complete and utter lack of sound. Pure, strange, and beautiful silence. Not a breath of wind. The depth of the darkness and the absolute stillness of the moment were unlike anything I had ever experienced before. The big lake before me was completely motionless, like a massive sheet of glass. I could feel my heart beating in my chest.

That's when I started noticing them.

Hundreds of lights that looked like they were shining up from the water appeared in one place on the surface of the lake. Then I noticed them in another place. Suddenly, I realized they were everywhere I looked, literally covering the entire lake. At first glance, I was completely confused. I had no idea what I was looking at or where these lights were coming from. Then I slowly lifted my chin and eyes to the sky. Time stopped. The lights I was seeing on the surface of the lake were the reflections of the millions of stars that lit up the night sky! As I looked up, I was in absolute awe. Immediately, the air escaped from my lungs in a gasp and exhale so deep I'll never forget it. My mouth dropped wide open as I gazed wide-eyed at the scene above my head. I had never seen anything close to that many stars shining at once. They completely blanketed the night sky. My mind wrestled to embrace the incomprehensible majesty, fullness, and expansiveness of what I was staring at.

There, in the divine stillness, on that dark, moonless August night, I saw the full stellular band of the Milky Way in spectacular clarity as it stretched from one point of the horizon to the other. As I cast my gaze across my surroundings, I saw millions of other stars I never even knew existed. The dizzying magnificence and beauty of this moment shook me to my core. I wondered, *How is it possible that this canopy and masterpiece of infinity sits above our heads every single night? How has this scene not provided more of the deeper answers about life to humanity?* In that moment of awe and wonder, millions of new questions filled my head about life, meaning, and purpose. This was the beginning of a beautiful journey to the answers.

From that moment on, no matter what place I was at in my life or what personal struggles I was going through, those big questions never left my mind. During my early teen years,

I painfully watched my parents separate a few times and eventually get divorced. After I graduated from high school, my family barely had enough money for me to go to college, and I was actually evicted from my college apartment sophomore year because my parents couldn't afford to help me pay my rent. Through sheer willpower, loans, and a lot of hard work, I did find a way to pay for school, complete my degree, and graduate. After graduation, I started life like many others, with no money and a heavy amount of college debt. But I used my business degree to get a job and started at the bottom of the finance industry. I worked extremely hard for long hours to build a clientele from nothing, all while making little or no money. At the same time, I was working on building my business, I fell in love and got married, and my wife and I had our first child, a healthy baby girl. We heartbreakingly lost a pregnancy to a miscarriage a year later, but like so many others, we grieved and when the time was right continued forward and had our second child, a healthy boy.

During all this time, through the ups and downs of life, the initial existential questions I'd asked about the nature of life never left my mind. The more I achieved, the more these deep, complex questions about life begged to be answered. This happened because the more I accomplished, the more I kept expecting to feel some sense of inner peace and ease. Yet what was happening was actually the exact opposite. The more I accomplished or accumulated, the more pressured and the more miserable I felt. So miserable, in fact, that I was losing my energy and zest for life. The importance of getting clarity on the path to true happiness, peace of mind, and success, whatever that was, became more vital to me than ever before.

In 2002, at the age of thirty-five, my questioning about life, purpose, and meaning had intensified to a tipping point. I had checked many of the boxes that mainstream culture tells us will bring happiness but still wasn't feeling the sense of fulfillment I desired. This made me cantankerous, unsettled, and at times depressed. There had to be a reason I was feeling empty rather than fulfilled by what I had or was working toward. Scared and starting to feel very hopeless, I anxiously and desperately wondered, "Why? What is it in the core of a person that gives them the ultimate sense of peace? If the wonderful things I already created in my life aren't providing me with a feeling of well-being, what will it take? Why do some people experience consistent success, happiness, and contentment in their lives, while so many others consistently deal with a lack of fulfillment, anxiety, and ongoing despair? How can I develop a mindset of faith, confidence, and positivity at every twist and turn and challenge of life? How does one find purpose and true creative success?"

In one pinnacle moment of utter desperation, I raised my hands up to the sky, got on my knees, and directly and urgently said to life, the universe, or any God that would listen, "I'm ready to know. Please show me what this life is all about! Please help me understand the meaning of it all." My questions emerged from a deep fear of more misery and a profound yearning for the answers to life. But on the other hand, my fearless desperation to know was beyond anything I'd ever felt before. I was ready to give up everything. I asked for it all, took a deep breath, and then released my questions like throwing a letter in a bottle into the ocean.

I was so drained at this point that after my hopeless moment of pleading I let go of any expectation that I'd ever learn or receive an answer in this lifetime. I did my asking, exhaled, then simply went back, exasperated, into my daily life.

I had no idea what would happen next. I was completely unaware that in that moment of intense asking, I was finally ripe and ready for some new, profound insights. I had finally opened myself up to receive the full magnetic force of universal wisdom. What I experienced is divine timing, a point where something occurs only when the exact conditions are right. In my case, the last condition occurred when my will to know finally exceeded my fear of knowing.

Two weeks after asking those deep questions, the answers to a lifetime of questioning began to flood my awareness. What I mean is that life seemed to be using almost every one of my daily experiences to send me a new insight or a new understanding. It started in a financial seminar I attended in 2002. The instructor discussed how investors create the experience of either a gain or loss in their investments based on all their preceding thoughts and decisions. He explained how those thoughts and decisions are in our control. Something about this resonated on a deep level with me. Suddenly, it hit me that this decision making was the exact process I was going through in my everyday reality, which was determining the quality of my experience of life! I had more power of choice than I had ever previously realized. This personal psychological understanding was not just about investment decisions in the financial markets but relatable to the experience of every part of my life.

In a flash of life-changing insight, I saw that I was building the conditions for my experiences in every moment of thought and action (consciously and subconsciously). My perception and reactions were shaping my experiences. This gem—that my perception was the key—revealed to me that I could shift the probabilities for how things unfolded in my life *once I became aware of how I was thinking*. I was simply astounded by this understanding.

Equally as mind-blowing, I realized that I had asked for this insight for years, and just two weeks earlier I had begged for answers in a state of readiness I had never felt before. Here it was, now, coming to me and showing up through every interaction in my daily life! What hit me was that this is how it all works. Life uses each moment and experience to serve us and help each of us grow in understanding and awareness based on our intentions. Life is intimately connected to us! But we won't see this connection or the universal knowledge it brings until we are ready for it. We must be ready for the awareness and the change it will bring. I finally got it! From that moment onward, I have gone into each day with a childlike wonder and excitement over how life is going to deliver me the clues and answers to my questions and creative intentions. What person, information, or experience was going to deliver the exact insight I was looking for?

Over the next six months, this state of profound peace produced a state of presence that enabled me to experience answers entering my awareness faster and faster. This continued to speed up until another massive moment of awakening occurred in December of 2002 that figuratively and literally blew my mind. I experienced a point of consciousness where the space between any question and its answer had completely collapsed. The best way to explain this is that I felt like the answers to so many of life's deepest questions were entering my mind before I even asked the questions. It was as if I opened up a portal in my mind at the top of my head, allowing endless wisdom to flow into it unabated. *Thinking had dissolved and all that was left was knowing.*

So much insight was revealed about how the dots connect between life, energy, purpose, and creation that it brought me to my knees in a state of profound humility that remains to this day hard to put in words. It took me well over a year to wrap my mind around both the magnitude and depth of what was revealed. This shift in consciousness left me with a vision and understanding of how life unfolds from almost every angle. The perfection and the inspiring infinite possibilities of all of life were revealed.

I was so incredibly humbled by the elegance and power of these insights that I have dedicated the rest of my life to honoring this wisdom by sharing it with others. My goal was, and continues to be, to be a good servant and deliverer of this grace. To let people know that this powerful wisdom is here right now, simply waiting to be realized. No résumé or requirement is necessary other than a curious and open mind. It is truly my honor to share my excitement that divine empowering truth is always as close to you as the whispering wind.

In the following couple of years, I wrote and had my first book published, *I AM: The Power of Discovering Who You Really Are*. *I AM* is dedicated to everything I came to understand about how life works from the inside out and the outside in. A few years later, I wrote another book, *Time in a Bottle: Mastering the Experience of Life*, which deals with how time plays a role in creating our intentions and dreams.

Along with writing and speaking, I began counseling and coaching individuals from every walk of life who were interested in applying this wisdom to all sorts of different challenges they were looking to overcome. I also received calls and emails from a significant number of college and professional athletes who told me they read *I AM* and immediately shifted their mindsets in a way that had a very profound effect on their performance and results. This led me to begin working with professional athletes in the same way I was working with business executives and individuals dealing with general life challenges. The results have been incredible. I've worked with athletes in all the major professional sports and with athletes in almost every sport at the collegiate level, as well as with many elite high school players. Several of the players' fascinating stories, including their breakthroughs and ultimate successes, are shared in this book.

THE KEY ATTRIBUTE OF SUCCESS

In the last two decades of teaching and coaching individuals to attain a more expanded state of consciousness and creation, I have discovered many critical aspects of the mindset of success. What remains consistent, and separates those who are happy, successful, and consistently achieving their goals from those who struggle with success or are just average rather than great, is their level of awareness of who they are and how they look at life.

The difference between those who create a life of flow and ease and those who face a life of constant setbacks, drama, and strife cannot be measured in terms of surface factors such as size, looks, strength, talent, or desire. It also has nothing to do with smarts or IQ. The distinction lies deep within the soul. It lies in how people see, believe, and act upon the truth of who they are. This truth is their beliefs and personal truths that start with "I AM."

"When I discover who I am, I'll be free."
—Ralph Ellison

Before this profound information entered my mind, I was struggling through life trying to figure it all out and discover more about who I am. Many moments of trial and error occurred before I came to see how life actually works in a synchronistic and serendipitous way with your identity. Not that there aren't challenges along the way. That's just life. But one of the simple and profound things I learned is that it's how you handle these challenges, based on who you are, that has the single biggest impact on your present and your future outcomes.

It is now my deepest honor to take these years of work and experience teaching people the process of supreme mental empowerment and share it with you. This book reveals exactly how you can embrace the same inner belief system and identity that creates breakthrough success for yourself. This is the exact step-by-step process of awareness that has worked for thousands of clients looking for empowering change. This ability is your birthright.

THE JOURNEY YOU ARE ABOUT TO TAKE

Invincible is laid out in a step-by-step format to help expand your consciousness and mental fortitude. You are embarking on a journey to understand how to work in complete harmony with life and its creative power. This wisdom is designed to take you to the place where you see the truth that anything is possible for you. It does not matter what circumstance you currently face. It does not matter what you dealt with in your upbringing or during any recent challenges. It does not matter what means you have or don't have. It does not matter what you have done or haven't done in your life. All that matters is that in this moment you have an open mind and a strong desire for change. You have to be willing to accept new information and reflect on and challenge some of the previous ways you have looked at yourself and life. These are the foundational first steps of positively changing your reality.

Expanding your awareness is like cleaning out your computer and updating its software so it runs smoother and faster with no risk of crashing. We don't realize how much our thoughts and perceptions clog our minds and slow down our performance. Overthinking and second-guessing ourselves can be energy draining, time-consuming, and a great burden on our souls. When this happens, it can keep us feeling incapable, stuck, and unable to move to the creative experience and results we really want.

Self-awareness is the ultimate cleanser and "software upgrade" for the operating system of the mind. It is the best way to expand the expression of your magnificent soul. Being open to learning is the best way to position yourself to receive priceless insight and the answers to your deepest questions.

THE INVINCIBLE MINDSET

With an invincible mindset, you have such a clear understanding of the limitless potential within you that no negative thoughts, challenges, or failed attempts can ever impede you or the respect and love you have for yourself. This mindset only knows one direction, and that is forward with every ounce of energy possible. In this state, you have a deep faith in how life is working with you. You ask yourself, "How could anything I experience be without purpose or meaning?" Instead of resisting any experience of life, you follow a more efficient path that involves a state of acceptance and a sense of curiosity and inquiry. You ask, "Why is this happening? What is this experience here to teach me?"

The other key to this invincible state of mind comes from a deep comfort with your identity. Because of your new self-confidence and respect for who you are, there is no denial of truth or wall of protection between you and what needs to be understood. Because you are open to insight, wisdom is attained more quickly, and your intentions materialize at a much faster pace. Each person's journey is different, so some take longer to learn lessons than others. However, when you have a deeper trust in life and how it works, the challenges you face have less of a negative impact on you. This is critical because your outlook is the greatest influence on your next experience. Knowing the most effective way to deal with what's happening in your life and how to generate an optimal, masterful response is one of the true keys to it all. This is how you ensure you get as many green lights as possible as you travel the road of life.

NEXT-LEVEL MINDFULNESS AND WHY IT MATTERS

In popular culture, mindfulness is generally defined as a state of presence and awareness of one's feelings and thoughts, and a nonjudgmental attitude about what is happening in the moment. Instructors usually teach that it can be achieved through breathing exercises or meditation.

The definition of mindfulness in this book expands on that definition. Next-level mindfulness is a state of presence where you are acutely aware of what is going on around you. In each situation you are able to either trust what's happening or connect the dots and see purpose and meaning as they relate to your ultimate intention. This automatically produces a nonjudgmental state of observance. In this balanced state you can see deeper into each situation and exactly what it needs. Next-level mindfulness is also a state of self-awareness where you can see how your thoughts and emotions have a direct impact on what is unfolding before you.

What worked thirty years ago, twenty years ago, or even ten years ago may not work today. To stay on the cutting edge, you are challenged to adopt new ways of seeing and responding to how life currently works. You must be in tune with the state of "what is" in life. In this ultracompetitive world, next-level mindfulness is the difference maker that puts you at the top of your game and mentally ahead of the rest. When you attain this level of mindfulness, your presence, focus, and ability to respond are always at a very high level, leaving little that the outer world can do to surprise you or throw you off-balance. The mind of a true master of reality is surprised by nothing.

> "If you correct your mind, the rest of your life
> will fall into place."
> —Lao Tzu

THE STRUCTURE OF THIS BOOK

This book is separated into three main sections and is structured in a step-by-step format. Please resist any urge to move ahead or out of order when you first read the book. Each step offers a critical understanding that is required to enhance the impact of the concepts in the next chapter. The purpose is to imbue you with the full understanding of both the intention of life, and the process of life and how it unfolds. When you embrace this insight, you will find the clarity and self-assurance that lead you to an invincible state of mind.

Part One: Self-Awareness

Step one: Step one offers the understanding of the main intent of life, how you directly connect to the universe of infinite potential, and how you are a part of this divine creative intent. This step reveals the co-creative nature of your relationship to life or the universe. It brings you to the understanding of how this co-creative nature affects your life and positively relates to your energy and what you are constructing for your life in every moment. Step one also explains the impact and quality of your energy and state of mind and how they affect your awareness, choices, and results.

Step two: With a true realization of the infinite potential that is life, you are ready to learn how the experiences of your past were created. Step two explains exactly how your identity has come together to shape who you have been, as demonstrated through the sum of your genetics, nurturing, perception, choices, and actions up until this moment.

Step three: This step builds on the understanding of step two to show you how in the same way you created parts of your past, you create your present and the probabilities for your future experiences. Step three reveals how your ego works with your truth to create your reality. In this step, I explain how thought, belief, and intention come together in this moment to influence your energy and actions. Understanding how your core beliefs (your "I AM . . ." statements) drive your ego's perception, reaction, and decisions is a key part of the motivation to enact real change.

Step four: Once you understand how your ego gets its instructions for action, you are ready for step four, which reveals how this power to create is often constrained by beliefs you've held that have limited your self-worth and what you believe is possible for you. These concepts (good and bad) affect personal growth and may have been embedded in your subconscious for years, potentially for generations. These are the hidden thoughts that have kept you from releasing the full creative power within you. In step four, you learn how to dissolve these limitations.

Part Two: Breakthrough

Step five: Step five builds on step four's momentum of unlimited possibility by offering how to liberate your soul and take on a new way of looking at who you are. This step of awareness unveils the power of self-acceptance, respect, and love. It reveals the path to personal freedom and the key to dissolving mental limitations and fears.

Step six: This step takes the freedom of the self-worth and potential you discovered in step five and shows you how to embrace it, accept it, and put it into action in your life. This is the step where you're guided through the process of embracing the mindset of infinite possibilities and you learn how to use the power of personal declaration (or the power of "I AM") and step into your new identity. It is about realizing how this authentic declaration propels you toward your dreams and desires.

Part Three: Next-Level Mindfulness

Step seven: Once you've learned how to create your experiences each day with a more empowered and optimistic perspective, you can turn to step seven, which is about being prepared to counter any destructive negativity you may encounter each day as you demonstrate the new you. This step teaches you how to be prepared for any challenge or test you come up against. Learning how to master any setbacks or tests you encounter as you wind on down the road of life is a crucial part of being invincible of mind.

Step eight: In this final step, you put together all you've learned. This is where I offer you the mindset of infinite potential and show you how to live successfully and joyfully in a state of flow and magical faith—in yourself and in life!

THE HEART AND SOUL OF THIS BOOK

A major intent of this book is to present you with a clear understanding of how life and everything in it connects with you and supports you. This book aims to leave you with no doubt about your power to choose how to experience life and about what you can accomplish. It's designed to help you become a victorious warrior of life and a master of the workings of your mind.

Many people in today's culture of instant gratification want quick answers to big questions. However, real wisdom and power come from an open mind and critical contemplation that reveals how you arrive at the answers you seek. It's the difference between getting the answer to one big math problem and learning exactly how an equation comes together and works so you can solve any equation or problem you encounter for the rest of your life. As Lao Tzu said, "Give a man a fish, you feed him for a day. Teach a man to fish, and you feed him for a lifetime."

Invincible is a manual of self-discovery. What you learn in these pages can be applied over and over along your entire journey of life. This book is a map revealing the power of who you can be. A blueprint that shows you that what you are worthy of and capable of creating for yourself is greater and more believable and achievable than you may have ever imagined.

The definition of the word *invincible* is "incapable of being overcome, conquered, or defeated." This quality is attributed to one who has an unwavering spirit and persistence in the face of any opposition, fear, or difficulty. It is my hope that with this sacred knowledge nothing will stop you from fully experiencing and expressing the joy of who you really are. This is peace. May your life flow freely and without fear or hesitation as you strive to achieve and experience all you dream is possible. May those you connect with feel the love of your expanded soul, liberated spirit, and indomitable will. May you be an inspiration in the world to all who know you as they benefit from your courageous journey to happiness, fulfillment, peace, and invincibility of mind!

The Light

I want the light
The light that liberates my soul.
I don't care what it reveals
As long as it makes me whole.

I want the light
The light that sets me free
From the pain I've long carried.
Finally relieved to be me.

I want the light
The light that dissolves my fear
Leading me into every moment
Open to more love than I can bear.

I want the light
The light that unveils my power.
I'm ready for a new destiny
For this is my true hour.

PART ONE

SELF-AWARENESS

REALIZING YOUR
INFINITE POTENTIAL

How You Are Connected to the Universe

Though my soul may set in darkness, it will
rise in perfect light; I have loved the stars too
truly to be fearful of the night.

—Sarah Williams

The vastness, beauty, and depth of the cosmos are trying
to tell us something. There is a beautiful mystery the
universe is working to unveil. Don't bother measuring
what you see. Don't try to rationalize it. Don't fear its depth.
Simply marvel. Marvel at the incomprehensible infinity and
perfection of it all. Who among us has not looked up on a
dark, moonless night and stood astonished at the miraculous
display they see above their heads? Who hasn't gazed across

a canopy of stars in the sky and wondered about what it all means? To think too deeply or to try to quantify a puzzle—or rather a masterpiece—so large causes a wiggle and a boggle in the mind. Your head can tend to recoil as the limits of how you look at life get stretched, pushed, and inspired to a new, unlimited perspective.

Philosophers, scholars, poets, mathematicians, scientists, physicists, and religious leaders over the centuries have all struggled to understand the meaning of it all. Yet what we keep finding as we look farther and farther into deep space is more and more manifested possibilities. The deeper we look, the more we find. Creation simply never ends.

The inescapable conclusion of the cosmos is that infinity is the truth of life.

THE REALITY OF INFINITE EXPRESSION

The way life or the universe demonstrates or validates the truth that it is infinite is by the awesome creative demonstration of the never-ending unfolding of infinite possibility. To do exactly what the universe is doing in every single moment—to be it. Depending on your spirituality or paradigm of accepted understanding, this awe-inspiring expression could be defined as God, Source, Brahman, or Universal Consciousness. As a collective consciousness, we are continually observing, revealing, and examining the reality of this energy and these never-ending possibilities. We are discovering them both in our lives and in the cosmos as we are examining them in a way we never have before. Life is consistently demonstrating through the expression of nature, human creativity, and the stars that the possibilities of what can be created are endless.

> "Emptiness which is conceptually liable to be mistaken for nothingness is in fact the reservoir of infinite possibilities."
>
> —D. T. Suzuki

Here's where it becomes important to connect the dots. If life is continually demonstrating the truth of infinite possibility and each of us is a part of this universe, then each one of us is endowed with that same power of infinite possibility, or rather the same ability for endless creation. Therefore, you are an unlimited creator of the experience of your life.

LIFE'S CONNECTION TO YOU

The first step on your journey to an empowered mindset is the understanding that life's core intention is to create infinitely. This is the fundamental starting point. "I AM that I AM"—a phrase referenced for thousands of years in religious texts as God's answer when asked, "Who are you?"—says it all. That's why you find creation everywhere you look.

Whether you look from a scientific, religious, or spiritual perspective, creation just keeps going and going uncontained.

You are a part of the universe and therefore a part of creation. The part that makes you uniquely human is a thinking, contemplating, self-reflecting, creative mind. As such, each day you are expressing who you are ("I AM . . .") based on *your* intentions. What you may not have fully realized yet is that life is in a moment-by-moment co-creative relationship with you and your intentions. The way life connects to you is by elegantly supporting you in creating whatever it is you intend to see, experience, and achieve. Life does this by working to bring about every condition required to increase the probability of your intention manifesting.

Your intent is the same as life's: to create in the continual effort to be. An experience of heartbreak, a discord or challenge in your life, and a time when you didn't get what you want are all part of the universe offering you something connected to one of your deeper intentions or goals. The question is, What are you truly intending to experience on this journey?

Life is bound to you to help you continually close the gap between what you intend to create and what you believe is true, consciously or unconsciously.

Life will consistently bring you the people, places, and events (or conditions) that will increase the probability that you create the experience that you believe is true or life will work to effectively shatter any lack of awareness (ignorance) that has kept you from your goal or intention. This is how powerful and unconditionally loving and supportive the connection is between life (God, the universe, Source) and you.

What's really interesting is that many people don't even know what they really believe is true or possible for themselves, or what is driving and creating their daily experiences. Many are also unaware of how their beliefs may be causing repeated suffering and additional time suffering.

One of the most significant steps in elevating your mindset is becoming aware of how what you believe about yourself influences both what you experience every day and how you experience it. The experiences you are co-creating with life can be either positive or negative. It all depends on what you believe is true. If you have a negative and fear-driven outlook on life, the probability increases that a negative experience will manifest for you. If you have a faithful and positive outlook, the probability shifts to a positive outcome. In working with thousands of people over the last twenty years, I have seen that this process occurs without fail. Every person is going through a process of shaping and manifesting certain thoughts, feelings, and experiences in order to validate the deeply held truths they have about themselves and life. Life is divinely connected to you in a way that helps you experience this validation.

YOU DID THE BEST YOU COULD

You cannot consciously cause what you don't know you are causing. Therefore, there is no value in feeling bad about past choices, actions, and responses when you did not know any better. Much of the inertia of your energy and the arc of your life path may have started generations before you. There is also no value in feeling bad about the past when you thought you knew better but felt you didn't do better. This is also a trap of mind. More about this will be revealed in future chapters.

> **You did the best you could at any past moment in time. If you could have done better, you would have.**

If you fear making mistakes or you work to avoid being vulnerable, you will block the process of self-reflection that offers the self-understanding that explains past actions and results. Preventing self-reflection (awareness) will only keep you stuck in a state of ignorance. This is why allowing yourself to potentially "fail" at times by being vulnerable and trying your best is so critical to becoming more aware of how to create your future. Life experiences allow you to understand yourself at a deeper level and lead you to make smarter, more efficient choices now, from this moment forward!

Seeing how every moment of life is working *with you* is the real meaning of "waking up." Next-level mindfulness is about being acutely aware that life is 100 percent tapped into what you believe is true and how much you intend to experience that truth. It is about understanding that life meets you with every resource to help you remove ignorance, gain awareness, and manifest your desires. It is here to help you become aware of how to align your core truths with what you say you really want to experience.

THE INTENT OF ALL ENERGY

To really understand how life meets you with a consistent stream of circumstances, you must have a fundamental understanding of energy and its impact on your mind, perception, and reactions. Realizing how life's energy organizes and influences the conditions that shape your life is a big part of learning how to *consciously* create what you experience.

Everything in your universe is made up of energy. It is the binding force behind all the matter in the known universe. As Albert Einstein famously concluded, "Energy cannot be created or destroyed; it can only be changed from one form to another." If energy cannot be created or destroyed, it is infinite. If energy is infinite, so are the creative ways and forms in which it expresses itself in the endless combinations of protons, neutrons, and electrons of the atoms that make up what you encounter every day. This energetic cycle of creative expression is always evolving, adapting, and changing in order to unfold, expand, and express infinitely. This is the intent and inertia of the movement of energy into matter and the moment-by-moment process of the evolution of life.

In my previous book, *Time in a Bottle*, I explained this idea by using Einstein's famous formula for how energy infinitely transforms into matter, $E = mc^2$ (energy = mass × the speed of light squared), and replacing the speed of light squared (c^2) with I for "intention."

Nothing can catch or pass the speed of light. That is why Einstein squared it in the equation. He concluded that this speed is the one thing that remains constant in the process where energy becomes matter in the infinite universe. In the same respect, nothing is faster than a thought that emerges in your mind. Thoughts seem to travel at the speed of light or happen instantaneously. We cannot get in front of a thought; we can only do so with another thought. Thought inspires our intention. Our intention determines exactly where we direct our attention and actions.

Where you put your attention determines a great deal of how your experiences of life come together. Observation (also known as attention) that is driven by intention causes the wave of formless universal energy to collapse and become an actual particle of matter on the smallest detectable scale. This was confirmed by the famous and groundbreaking double-slit experiment where quantum physicists found that attention or the act of observing (consciousness) determines when energy or a wave of infinite potential collapses and transforms into a single possibility as an actual detectable piece of matter. The implication is that your attention has a major impact on how things come together for you. Therefore, it makes sense to insert *I* for "intention" into the equation to reveal a *psychological or metaphysical version* of Einstein's formula for his theory of relativity for how creation unfolds.

Rewriting the equation, we get $E / I = M$, meaning the formula for creation is

Energy divided by Intention equals Mass.

In the metaphysical or spiritual paradigm, the way of expressing Einstein's scientific equation is

Infinity divided by thought = matter.

In the religious paradigm, the way of expressing the equation would be

God divided by creation = life.

Or, as it has been demonstrated since the beginning of human curiosity,

Thought becomes reality.
Mind becomes matter.
"I" becomes "AM."

Everything in existence has emanated from either an intention (force/counterforce) or a conscious human thought that became an intention put into action. This is true for everything from inanimate inorganic objects to plants and animals to human beings. A thought is a single finite possibility manifested from a sea of infinite possibility, a drop of water pulled from the ocean of potential into existence.

HOW LIFE EXPRESSES THE POSSIBILITIES

To see this powerful display of energy moving to expand creation, you simply need to look around your world. Currently there are over 18.5 million known species of plants and animals on the planet. Each year scientists discover over 18,000 completely new species! It is the same with the endless number of stars that sit above your head every night. The Hubble Space Telescope, launched in 1995, was miraculously able to discover over 100 billion new galaxies in deep space. However, in view of the 2021 launch of the new James Webb Space Telescope, the staggering estimation is that the number of discovered galaxies will increase to over 200 billion! For some crazy context, our galaxy, the Milky Way, is estimated to contain 100 to 400 billion stars! The number of new galaxies being discovered by this new telescope, along with the astronomical (pun intended) number of stars within them, is truly a mind-blowing figure.

The inescapable reality is that the expression of life is infinite. Life's main intention is to express these infinite possibilities and the finite experience of these *infinite possibilities*.

You are an expression of these possibilities, a creator of possibilities, and one who observes and experiences possibilities.

Every aspect of life (and every living thing) is constantly working toward the persistent continuation of its expression. Therefore, the main intention of all creation is survival. That is why the plant bends toward the sun for energy or the animal changes its color to adapt to and camouflage itself in the surrounding landscape. That is why one of the strongest natural urges for human beings is procreation.

The intent of the energy behind all matter is to persist and continue to express itself for as long as possible.

Life most effectively expresses itself through creative distinction. That is why thousands of new species emerge each year. That is why creativity drives life. That is why the human species finds a sense of fulfillment and self-identity in traveling to a new place; learning new information or a new skill; developing a new relationship; being part of a larger group; and trying different clothing styles, tattoos, social media expressions, jewelry, art, or any other manifestation that brings distinction, reflects growth, and attracts attention by saying:

I exist.

I matter.

I AM.

THE CHALLENGE OF FINDING MEANING IN TODAY'S WORLD

The way we experience our identity in society has dramatically shifted in the internet and social media age. For most of human history, the focus of everyday living was on pure survival. The ability to eat, drink, find shelter, and procreate was the main driving intent. But how individuals find meaning and define themselves has radically changed over the last hundred years or so. With all the modern conveniences, identity and purpose are no longer predominantly rooted in survival or in escaping the threat of extinction. Finding water, food, and shelter or being connected to a larger community is no longer the consistent daily priority for a majority of the population in first world countries. Instead, personal motivation and intention (energy) have shifted and are now predominantly focused on finding fulfillment by developing a vocation of interest; working toward experiencing a certain dream, creative goal, or desire; expressing oneself; and ultimately finding meaning in life and feeling at peace with oneself.

This search for a new way of living and expressing who we are is at the heart of the current mental health crisis. Millions are having a hard time finding meaning, connection, and purpose. Many are now chasing fulfillment by way of instant self-gratification, political movements, accumulation of material possessions, unbalanced and unhealthy fixations on a cause, or social media presence. The results of these new attempts to feel fulfilled aren't great. While some of these efforts work, many do not, because they lack the deep purpose that comes from truly connecting with others or adding value to the community or world.

That is why there is so much unrest in today's more disconnected society. So many who have lost hope have defaulted to simply getting mired in the negativity of the online world or in the images on their smartphone screens. People go online or on social media to feel more connected and to find meaning, a voice, or a sense of value. But as a result, they often become even more frustrated and disillusioned.

This trend has led to a major increase in anxiety and depression in many people who have yet to find real fulfillment in who they are. At the same time, many of the same people are being bombarded with images on social media of the lie of what it looks like to have a "better" or "perfect" life. Not a good combination. I've talked with so many teens and young adults about this very issue. In this environment, it can be difficult for people to understand how to feel good about themselves, connect with others, and be optimistic about the future.

When your soul is not fulfilled, your ego (the part of you tasked with validating your existence) searches for something to do to find meaning or change your state of mind. You can end up feeling the need to make impulsive and unhealthy choices or to use drugs or indulge in other forms of destructive vices to escape anxiety, general negativity, or feelings of hopelessness.

However, if you have been in these troubling states or have had negative thoughts about your future, know that there is a way out of this suffering. There is a path to gaining back control of your mind and creating new possibilities for yourself. The answer is found in the process of self-realization. Through a new understanding of who you are, a new way of looking at the world emerges. This new perspective, which reveals your worth and how much you matter, can change everything for you. In this new state you see that each moment holds nothing but possibility for you.

THE IMPORTANCE OF RELENTLESS OPTIMISM

To condition your mind to create the life you desire, you must protect your mindset from negative and limiting perspectives. These include the negative thoughts of others and your own tendency to adopt a negative outlook. The next-level results you desire for your life can only be created and experienced by a consistently positive mind that is open to change and ripe to embrace success.

An important takeaway from step one is that you are part of an infinitely creative universe. You are here to create and express. The key to how many of these possibilities you can see, believe in, and act toward for yourself will depend on your level of self-worth and the quality of your mindset. *The enlightened path is to develop an authentically strong optimistic and positive mind and protect it at all costs.*

Those who have fulfilling lives of flow and synchronicity come from a place of mind where there is no doubt that anything is possible. The question is not *if* they are going to make what they want to happen for themselves, but *how*. They are hyperfocused on the information they need to get closer to their goal. Therefore, they stay open to learning and they do not let destabilizing emotions or any outside noise or negative energy distract them from their focus. Energetic balance is key.

HOW YOUR PERCEPTION AFFECTS THE QUALITY OF YOUR STATE OF MIND

The energy that moves through you is working for your self-expression and creating your experiences of life based on your beliefs and what you feel you need to do to survive. Everyone else's energy is doing the exact same thing. How satisfied you are with this self-expression and your resulting experiences shows up in your state of mind. Your state of mind determines the polarity of your energy and the intensity of your emotions. Therefore, your perception can have a positive or negative effect on your energy and emotions. Or your perception may produce no effect on your state of mind and your energy may remain neutral, meaning no emotion will result. Understanding how your state of mind can be affected one way or another is essential to self-mastery.

There are three ways of perceiving your reality that determine your energy and state of mind:

1. **How you interpret the current status of your world:** This aspect of perception involves the people around you, the situations and events you experience, and how you respond to them.

2. **How you perceive yourself and your circumstances:** This is about how much your current experiences match and satisfy who you think you are or who you think you should be.

3. **How you interpret and respond to other people's energy:** This refers to the energy that comes directly at you each day from interactions, expressions, and conversations with other people and how you react to it.

The state of your energy determines the quality of the energy you emit, and therefore is a critical determining factor in how you construct your experience. This is important because your state of mind determines your level of clarity and objectivity. A diluted, emotional, and imbalanced state of mind leads to diluted reactions and choices. Undesired outcomes become more likely as life reflects back this lack of awareness. The clearer and more balanced the mind, the more clear, powerful, and aligned your choices and reactions become. Making more aware choices increases the probability that you will experience what you want or desire.

Consider how a negative state of mind can influence you

and cause you to make an undesired situation worse: If you resist the state of your job, your relationship status, the current state of politics, or any other situation you encounter, this resistance will create negative energy to a certain degree. The more resistance, the more negative energy. The more negative energy, the more emotional you will become. The more emotional you are, the less empowered you are to take your life in the direction you desire.

The point is not that you shouldn't disapprove of any of the events of your world that are not in harmony with your value system. Rather, the point is to be aware of how resistance to any current truth of life can have a negative impact on your mind. This can throw you off-balance and prevent you from gaining the clarity and power needed to move the needle in a more positive direction regarding what you desire. The most empowered, peaceful, and accomplished people in the world are hyperaware of how the energy of the world can negatively affect the power of their minds. They simply don't let it affect them and their focus.

All information in the world is neutral until you sense, perceive, and interpret it.

Two people can have drastically different experiences of and reactions to the same information or event. For example, the experience of learning who won a political race will produce different reactions for those on each side of the political spectrum. Different people will respond differently based on whether it's hot or cold out. Whether it rains or snows. Which sports team wins. What laws change in a country. What stock goes up or down. In each of these circumstances, one person will be uplifted by the outcome, and another will be unhappy about it. (Those who don't care about the event or information will have no emotional reaction.) Within these thousands of experiences people are having, there will also be different levels of reactions and resulting emotions. In one sense this realization is so incredibly powerful and in another it seems so simple. The takeaway and massive nugget of empowerment is that you control the impact of any information that hits your senses. It is all neutral until you decide which way it matters and how much it matters.

Acceptance of the simple fact that any undesired world circumstance simply *is*, or exists, is the empowered path. You always hold the power to decide how any circumstance in the world affects you.

It's only human to have an initial negative reaction to an undesired result in your life, a tragic event, or a terrible circumstance in the world. The question is, How much does the event have to affect your mind and how long does your reaction have to linger? To live in the most empowered way, however, is to embrace what is true as fast as you can in order to retain clarity and mental balance. How you reflect upon yourself and benchmark what is happening against your beliefs and expectations can have a major impact on your state of mind.

If you are resistant to the circumstance or how it affects you, you will experience mental disharmony and your state will shift to the negative side of the emotional spectrum. If you are enjoying a very pleasing new experience of who you are or what is happening in your world, a positive shift and an imbalance on the positive side of the emotional spectrum will occur. And if you are satisfied as you reflect on the past, the current moment, or your future, your energy will be in harmony and balance. You'll be at peace.

When it comes to your inner dialogue, the point is not that you shouldn't occasionally evaluate yourself and your life and strive for change. This is a common part of being human. The point is that you should be acutely aware of how negative self-reflection can be a trap for the unconscious mind that can quickly send your energy and state of mind down a slippery, destructive slope. This adds unnecessary time and suffering to your path. You don't ever want to be your own worst enemy.

The empowered mindset sees the perfection of this moment and the exact path that created it.

Every day, you are confronted with the energy of other people. This could be the energy, emotions, and interactions from family members, friends, clients, bosses, coworkers, significant others, or even strangers. Each of these interactions will immediately go through the perception, interpretation, and reaction cycle of your mind. The way you perceive these interactions and how you decide to let this energy affect you are critical. Learning to be more conscious of what has primarily been a subconscious process of allowing the surrounding energy to affect you is the beginning of a positive change in your experience and a critical part of becoming mentally invincible.

You can't physically see this energy, just as you can't see radio or satellite waves or a Wi-Fi signal. But you can feel this energy and its effects. Have you ever walked into a room where someone is down and depressed and physically felt their negatively charged energy on your mind and body? Have you ever been in a situation where someone was trying to sell you something or coerce you into doing something in a pushy way? Most likely, it repelled you or you felt like you needed to get out of the space, go home, and shower off the bad vibe. While these are more extreme examples, every day the world is coming at you with an energy that can drain you and mentally and physically wear you out, if you let it.

Certain people in your life, especially close relatives, actually count on you to take on their energy and react in a certain way. Because of a lifetime of interactions, you already have an expected role to play and a precedent has been set. The question is, Does that role serve you now? Do you want to receive your power back and to remain unaffected by the energy, approval, or manipulation from others? In many cases it only takes one comment from someone close to you to automatically affect or trigger you. The result is usually an immediate emotional and physiological reaction. The idea is to be so prepared and mentally ready regarding who you want to be now that nothing knocks you off-balance.

Acknowledging any past energetic effects on you from others is a massive first step in taking control of your mindset. This energetic effect may have been going on for years without you realizing it consciously. Some friends and relatives can be so draining to be around that there is a term for them: "energy vampires." These kinds of people often need to vent so much negative energy and can require so much attention that you feel like they are draining the energy out of your body.

For example, if your father says something negative or offensive about your significant other, your blood pressure is likely to rise, and the inconceivable nature of the comment will cause resistance and a surge of negative emotion that you will have to work to contain. (Deep breaths will probably be a good first step.)

Encountering an irate person while driving or in line at the grocery store has the potential to affect you as well, possibly putting your mind on high alert. If you let this happen, adrenaline starts to flow, and you become susceptible to negative emotions and reactions, which your mind initiates as a defense mechanism when it detects a threat.

In another scenario, you read an Instagram comment or a tweet that runs completely counter to what you believe is true or think is appropriate for your world. You immediately get angry and charged up and begin to write all sorts of replies and counterarguments to the comment. You ultimately feel drained by the interaction.

These are just a few everyday examples of how your daily interactions have the potential to throw you off-balance and put you into a fight-or-flight mode. When you're in this disrupted, unbalanced state, you can't effectively create or initiate thoughts and actions that lead to positive change. Instead, your state of mind becomes focused only on protecting yourself and your values from a perceived attack.

Becoming a master of your reality is partly about being aware of any negative energy and the impact it can have on your sacred state of mind, and partly about being prepared to deal with this energy in a way that serves your desire to cultivate your mind for success and happiness.

HOW YOUR STATE OF MIND AFFECTS YOUR RESULTS

Your state of mind, along with the quality of energy it produces, is the moment-to-moment output of your "truth," which directly influences the creation of your reality. *This is exactly why it is so critically important that you protect the quality of your state of mind at all times.* A mindset of infinite potential and invincibility depends on it.

The quality of your energy determines how you *feel* in any given moment, and this determines the polarity of your energy and emotions. Emotions reveal the truth of how you feel. Emotions are energy in motion (*E*-motion), and they are a result of any energetic imbalance. When this imbalance becomes too large, the mind then seeks to vent the imbalance (emotions) in the attempt to get back to balance.

The idea to remember is that emotional states do not produce top-level results. They produce choices and actions from a clouded, unfocused, impatient mind. Examples of two different emotional states are blissful arrogance and fearful need. Both will create choices from a limited and nonobjective state of mind. Both are highly narrow and subjective states that have the potential to produce blind spots and pitfalls that can cause problems or set you back.

In blissful arrogance you're likely to think you can't lose the game, or you can't fail at business, or your significant other would never leave you no matter what you do. In fearful need you will likely try too hard as an athlete, creating more pressure; repel potential buyers in business; or overcontrol your significant other. The point being that any energy imbalance immediately starts to affect your mental clarity and severely dilutes the quality of your choices and responses. Highly emotional states of mind limit how well you can assess and perform in that moment. They limit how well you can create.

The state of calm confidence is much more balanced, clear, and objective. Choices and decisions made in this highly aware state have a much higher probability of being aligned with what you desire and what will move you toward your desired outcome. That's why a great piece of advice is to always wait a couple of hours before responding to an email or text that enraged you. You're much more likely to be in a clearer state of mind and much less likely to regret your response. In turn, you're more likely to communicate effectively. The most productive state of mind, which enables you to respond more quickly and effectively, is one of pure balance, also known as a state of complete peace.

All great athletes know this on some level. That's exactly where the saying "never too high, never too low" comes from in sports. It's all about the effort to find the magical state of balance or what is known as "the zone." The legendary basketball player Kobe Bryant certainly knew how to get into this state. In an interview some years ago, Kobe shared how he would get his mind ready for optimal performance. He said that for many years, "as psychotic as it seems" (in his own words), he would put headphones on before games and listen to the soundtrack from the horror movie *Halloween*. He explained that he did this to put himself in the most emotionless, and therefore focused, state possible. He prepared his mind to compete by associating the music with the masked, emotionless face and determination of the main character in the horror film. Kobe knew his mind had to be clear, balanced, and, most importantly, laser focused on the goal. He wanted to be in the most determined and undistracted state possible so he could use all his energy and talent to dominate on the court. The soundtrack to this movie is what put him in this highly focused state of mind. Because, as he said, when he's in that state, "You better run!"

Another interesting example from the world of sports involves the tennis great John McEnroe. McEnroe was one of the most legendary and dominant tennis players of the 1980s. Throughout his career he won seven individual and nine doubles Grand Slam titles and was ranked number one in the world. He was a mentally strong and feisty competitor his entire career. However, it is McEnroe's antics and behavior during many of his matches that make him an interesting study on managing mindset. Besides being a world-class player, McEnroe was known for his childish and emotional outbursts at the chair umpire during matches. He would argue points and yell endlessly at the referee about a bad or missed call. One of the many unbecoming things he shouted was the famous line, "You cannot be serious!" This caused jeers from the crowds, hefty fines, and a lot of damage to his reputation. But on closer inspection, there was a subconscious method to his madness.

Athletes cannot find their sharpest focus and presence when they are in an emotional state. Actually, no one can, whether they are an athlete or not. So there are two choices: find a way to not allow things to bother you or find a way to get the imbalance of energy—generated by your frustration—out of your system as efficiently and quickly as possible. Clearly, McEnroe allowed many things to bother him during play, including his own insecurities, his poor play at times, and the pressure of competition. However, he found a very boisterous and unconventional way of dealing with it. When the emotional buildup in his mind became too large, he vented the massive energy by yelling and screaming at the chair umpire before the next service point. This is what helped him get refocused. Such behavior would never be tolerated today, but releasing the buildup of negative energy from his mind allowed him to get balanced and clear once he was done with each tantrum. As a matter of fact, many people were mystified about his ability to shift from being violently upset and yelling out of control in one moment to concentrating and executing shots at a world-class tennis level in the next moment.

The answer to the mystery lies in the fact that the emotional system is designed to move energy out of us to help us get back to a greater state of awareness and clarity. Where there is clarity, there is focus and intuition. McEnroe may not have realized this on a conscious level, but the relentless competitor in him surely knew this on a subconscious level. Not until the last bit of excess energy and emotional imbalance was jettisoned from his mind through a snarky, vinegar-laced comment to the referee would he serve the ball. Bounce, bounce, comment, comment, bounce, comment, bounce, balance, clarity, bounce, serve!

When you are trying to achieve success at a very high level, energetic, mental, and emotional balance is imperative.

Any time you make choices from a mental place of need or fear, you are validating the need and fear. You are also acting from a limited view of what's possible. In other words, your response is expressing what you really believe to be true. But as you will learn as you progress through the steps of this book, what you believe to be true has the biggest influence over the way the circumstances of your life come together.

For example, in the case of McEnroe, if he served the ball or played the next point believing he was being cheated by the chair umpire, his mind and body would have worked to fulfill that belief subconsciously by the lack of a full concentration or effort. Ultimately, by way of a self-fulfilling prophecy, he would have lost. Incredibly, his unconventional way of clearing his mind got him back to enough optimism and focus to go on with the serve and ultimately win many of these matches. In 1984 alone, McEnroe set the tennis record for singles victories with an astonishing eighty-three wins and three losses. However, his behavior wasn't without karma. That year, he had a crushing defeat in the French Open finals to Ivan Lendl that included many of these outbursts. In his autobiography, McEnroe said he's never quite gotten over it.

When it comes to your life, how you manage your state of mind works exactly the same. If you are in a state of fear or need in your relationship, you will experience a host of problems, as you will always be on the edge of an imbalanced emotional state. Fear will shape your perception, and you will focus only on what you fear. This fear and need may push the other person away and fulfill the negative vision of what you believed to be true.

The same is true when it comes to business, your health,

or your career. How you shape the energy of your perception each day affects your emotions and state of mind. The quality of this energy then permeates every cell in your being. This determines whether you are creating or destroying the dreams you have for your life. In other words, your perception, which polarizes your energy (positive or negative), has an impact on how you experience time. Time, in this case, means how soon you begin to experience what you desire.

The more conscious you are of how your perception affects you and your decisions, the more *empowered* you are to contemplate and respond with the choices that most directly *serve* your intentions and dreams. On the other hand, a continued lack of awareness of your perceptions, reactions, and energy output will take you further away from what you want to experience. If you allow the way you perceive things to cause conflict and overwhelming emotions, it will restrict your awareness, causing you to make choices without clarity of mind. In other words, you will make decisions from a state of ignorance rather than a state of understanding.

THE FIRST STEP TO AN INVINCIBLE MIND

Step one in the process of learning the invincible mindset is to embrace infinite possibility and how life or the universe aims to help you uncover this truth. This step is also about understanding how your perception and energy and the energy of others can affect your state of mind and prevent you from realizing these great possibilities. This understanding is critical to your success. Your pivotal question, then, is "How do I change the way I perceive things so that my energy, state of mind, and the way I interact with life are most aligned with the future I want to experience?"

The answer to how you align your mindset with your dreams lies in the way you see who you are.

As mentioned earlier, your state of mind at any given moment always reveals what you believe to be true. Perception is therefore based on personal truth. *The sum of your personal truths about yourself and life is your identity.* Your identity is the foundation of your perceptions of yourself, the world, and your circumstances.

In over twenty years of private coaching sessions, I have had hundreds of discussions with clients about shifting how they look at themselves and the world. That shift is the basis for all positive transformation. Here is some actual dialogue from one of these conversations. While my client and I were discussing relationships in this example, this mindset shift can be applied to many aspects of life, including business success, peace of mind, and achievement of next-level results in sports.

ME: So you don't believe that finding lasting love is possible?
CLIENT: No, not a chance. Not after what I've been through.
ME: Tell me, have you ever looked up at the stars on a dark night somewhere away from the city lights?

CLIENT: Well, yes, when I was younger.

ME: What did you see?

CLIENT: A lot of stars!

ME: What does that tell you about space and the cosmos?

CLIENT: That it's big and vast.

ME: What's another word for that?

CLIENT: I don't know, endless?

ME: Keep going.

CLIENT: Boundless?

ME: Keep going.

CLIENT: Infinite?

ME. Bingo.

ME: Does *infinite* mean limited in possibility or unlimited in possibility?

CLIENT: Well, unlimited, I guess.

ME: You guess?

CLIENT: No, it means unlimited in possibility.

ME: Are you a part of this infinite universe of unlimited possibility?

CLIENT: Well, yes.

ME: Then that same potential that is expressed nightly in the trillions of galaxies that surround us is within you.

CLIENT: [In the voice of Jim Carrey from the movie *Dumb and Dumber*] So you're telling me there's a chance . . .

ME: That's funny. Yes! There is always the possibility for change and the reality you want emerging in your life. There is always the hope of what you desire happening. Infinite possibility surrounds you in every moment. This

58

is a critical door for you to open and walk through as a starting point for our work together.

CLIENT: OK, I'm listening, but if anything is possible, why can't I fly or play basketball in the NBA?

ME: OK, so wasn't flying around the world in airplanes impossible around two hundred years ago? How about soaring in hang gliders that have fans propelling them? And now there are wingsuits that enable people to fly down from mountains and airplanes, so we are getting closer and closer to flying being a reality. But that's not really your intention, anyway. Neither is playing in the NBA, or you would have trained to be an elite player in high school and then college. But, back to the point, is there anyone your age who has been through what you've been through in relationships, has found true love again, and is happier than they've ever been before? Yes, thousands and thousands of people. So let's stay focused and hopeful on that same possibility for you as well.

HOW YOU CHANGE YOUR RESULTS

The self-fulfilling nature of life is what causes you to look at life and act in a way that works to prove what you already believe to be true. Therefore, you are a prisoner of the limits of your thinking and beliefs only until your truth changes. That's why having an open mind is so critical to living from an invincible mindset and creating a fulfilling life. If you don't like the results you are currently experiencing and you want to change your experience to something better, then it's time to look within and change your truth and hence change your identity. It's time to change the way you look at who you are.

The creative force of life (or the universe) doesn't just deliver what you *want*, but rather seeks to serve you with what you currently *need* to see, know, and understand so you can more effectively create what you want. *Life will meet you with the precise awareness that helps you close the gap between what you say you want and who you believe you are.* This book in your hands is proof of that statement. You always have free will in how fast you embrace that awareness, demonstrate a new intent (behavior), and move toward your goals.

This information is designed to help you become more conscious of the truths that have run your life up until now and to help you learn to take more *conscious control* of the way you think and act going forward. It's the only way to break through to real, lasting change.

Once you have embraced the reality of infinite possibility and have realized how energy affects your state of mind and results, you are ready for step two in the process of building an invincible mindset. Understanding your identity and how it has affected your past behavior is a major step in this process. This awakened understanding allows you to consistently direct your thoughts and actions in a way that is more aligned with manifesting your deepest desires.

STEP 1 REFLECTION QUESTIONS

The purpose of the reflection questions in the first four steps of the book is to help you determine if your mind is resisting any newfound truths and identify what beliefs may be preventing you from moving to a more empowered and invincible state of mind. Answer yes or no to each of the following questions. If your current answer to any of the questions is no, use a journal, a sheet of paper, or your phone to write down *why* you currently feel this way. Refer to the notes you take here as you move through the rest of the steps in the book. The intent is that by the time you finish the book, you will be able to come back and answer every question with a genuine and emphatic yes!

1. Do you believe in a universe of unlimited and infinite possibilities?

2. Do you believe you have unlimited potential to create what you desire?

3. Do you believe that the universe is working with you to help you fulfill your truth?

4. Do you understand how your state of mind and energy affect your choices, actions, and reactions?

5. Do you believe you have ultimate control over your state of mind?

STEP 2

UNDERSTANDING YOUR IDENTITY

How Genetics and Environment Formed Who You Were—but Not Who You Are

> If you seek to understand the whole universe,
> you will understand nothing at all. But seek
> to understand yourself and you will under-
> stand the whole universe.
>
> —Druidic axiom

U nderstanding how your past has come together up to this moment is critical to creating a mindset of infinite potential. In step one, you learned that the force of life is working to help you express your unlimited nature. In step two, you will come to know how life has worked seamlessly to create your past experiences.

The first thing to realize is that your past does not have to influence your present or your future unless you allow it to have influence. One of the most exciting things about life is how everything can change for the better in this very moment. A big part of increasing the probability for this change is becoming fully aware of how your identity has played a role in creating your past. Why is this awareness so important? Because you can't change a process or a pattern affecting your life if you aren't aware that there's been a process or a pattern affecting your life.

Gaining this insight is liberating for two reasons. One, it gives you an understanding of a big reason for the decision-making, life path, and experiences of your past. And two, it's beyond exciting to realize that just as you have created a good portion of your past from a lot of unconscious thoughts and actions, you can create your future from an even more powerful place of understanding and awareness: from a *conscious* state!

When learning how you consciously create your experience of life, there is nothing that is more important than the understanding of your identity.

THE INFLUENCE OF YOUR IDENTITY

Your true identity, or the "I" of the powerful self-declaration "I AM," has been the driving force of how your life has unfolded. Your identity is the current reflection of your soul. Another way of explaining this is that your identity represents your level of consciousness. It represents every single truth you hold about who you are. These "truths" are what you believe is true about yourself regardless of what anyone else believes about you. They even include truths you hold that run counter to what you think and say about yourself.

For example, you may think or often say that you're a great boyfriend, girlfriend, or partner and that your relationship is solid. However, when it comes to your true identity, what matters is not what you think and say, but rather what you believe to be true on the deepest and most influential level of thought. If you are out of touch, you will most likely miss key signs of where your relationship is coming apart. Awareness helps you see this and change things before it's too late. Your level or lack of awareness is what actually produces the experiences, circumstances, and quality of the relationship. As far as life is concerned, it's only your deepest core truths ("I AM . . .") that determine the probability of how things will come together for you throughout your relationship.

What you believe is true is the single most important factor in the construction of your life from this moment forward.

You may think you are a top athlete on your college or professional team. The real driver of the process will always be the truth you hold about who you are. Again, it doesn't matter whether you look confident or what you say or feel. What matters is what you *believe* is true about who you are. This will determine how every sequence and play come together for you. Your truth will determine your level of ignorance or awareness of what needs to be improved in order to accomplish your goals. Any lack of awareness (or ignorance) will add to the time it takes you to achieve the success you desire.

In every case your core defining truths ("I AM . . .") rule your mind, your perspective, and the actions and reactions that shape what happens next. The more you believe yourself to be unlimited, the more stable, balanced, and opportunistic you feel. Some people have been called "old souls" or "wise souls." These individuals exhibit a more expanded awareness and a deeper sense of self that reflect a calmer, peaceful presence. The interesting thing is that this quality is based not on age but on the level of awareness the person exhibits. Many of these types of people seem to exhibit this expanded state of being from the day they are born.

When you see yourself as limited, unworthy, and small in terms of capability or opportunity, your perceived field or "bubble of possibilities" is much smaller than when you see yourself as worthy and define yourself in a way that includes many yet-to-be-discovered versions of yourself. The more you believe in yourself, the more possibilities you have available to you. As you learn more and more about the true nature of who you are, your bubble of possibilities expands dramatically. This view on life tends to produce more hope, more inspiration, and a more relaxed state of being.

A *limited* or smaller sense of self-worth can even show up in a person who is successful in one particular area of life. For example, an athlete whose identity is completely wrapped up in their success in their sport constantly feels that their identity is at risk in their next performance. This sets them up for a major crisis if their performance does not meet their expectations. The potential for crisis is the same for people in relationships who make their significant other their "whole world."

There are two major concerns in these cases. The first is the pressure that can arise from the need to keep validating one's identity in order to feel calm and secure. For example, the athlete will put too much pressure on performing rather than relaxing and letting their true talent shine. The person in the relationship will put too much pressure on their significant other in order to quell their own insecurities. Both scenarios have unintended negative consequences. The second problem is that people who put too much emphasis on the idea that only one way of life can define them generally fear who they will be without this identity. Any time fear dominates the mind, emotional imbalance, clouded decisions, and general panic are not far behind. When there is fear in the mind, destruction is a likely outcome. This is because all the thoughts and actions are being generated from the belief (truth) in what is feared. For example, a person who is insecure about their identity and sense of value might be fearful and think, *My partner is going to leave me*, or, *I am not going to make the team.*

On the other hand, those who are very happy and succeed in sports, relationships, or life have a more solid, confident, and *unlimited* view of their personal identity. Their view of themselves is vaster and more encompassing. They have a deeper faith in their ultimate survival. They are more relaxed and comfortable with themselves and know they will be OK.

As much as any athlete who is confident *thinks* they will succeed, one who has a more *unlimited* and stable identity *knows* they will ultimately achieve success. This keeps them very calm and focused in the moment, no matter what adversity they face. Athletes with an unlimited view of themselves and their abilities are very present and highly aware. Their natural talents and instincts lead to greater intuition, allowing them to act and react in a very productive way.

In any relationship a certain amount of self-confidence is critical for clarity and balance. It is also attractive to exhibit a cool, calm, and collected demeanor. Individuals who are more grounded in a solid sense of self are always highly aware of the tone of their relationship or keen and mindful at all times regarding where a deeper connection may need to be nurtured. They do not let fear or paranoia infect their thoughts or dictate how they act, because they trust that they will be OK no matter what happens with the relationship. This allows them to be fully authentic, vulnerable, and connected. Thus, they foster the tenets of true attractiveness and intimacy.

The bottom line is that when it comes to elevating your mind to a powerful creator of your intentions, you cannot be driven by need. You cannot be in a state of fear. You must trust who you are, no matter the circumstances, to keep the probability of success in your favor.

THE IMPACT OF YOUR UPBRINGING: NURTURE

Just as it's crucial to understand that your identity or sense of self (limited or unlimited) creates and affects your experiences in life, it's important to understand how your identity was formed in the first place. There are three major elements that work together to form your identity: upbringing, genetics, and personal experiences.

The first element, upbringing, is the way you have been nurtured. How your primary caregivers nurtured you and cultivated their relationship with you since your birth had a major impact on your sense of self. Your caregivers shaped your first interactions with your world and ultimately your sense of value. Were you left to cry in the crib for long periods of time? Did you receive the attention, food, diaper changing, and connection that cultivated a sense of safety and security? Your treatment left deep impressions and has influenced your perceptions of and reactions to certain situations and events in your life ever since.

How were your relationships with your parents, caregivers, or those you looked up to when you were a toddler or small child? Did you feel loved and protected? And equally important, how did you feel about the level of love and acceptance you received from your mother or father as a preteen and a teenager? How you held these relationships in your mind and what they represented in terms of your self-worth have been critical forces in your life, shaping your beliefs about yourself and your self-respect, self-worth, and self-love. These were the very first interactions that gave you a sense of who you are. It makes perfect sense that how you felt you were treated determined your self-worth or the lack of it. As a child, you simply had no other reference point. In many cases, your caregivers were the individuals who birthed you into existence. How could you not have been deeply influenced by the quality of these relationships?

These feelings and how they have caused you to reflect on yourself have turned into the choices, actions, and intentions you've demonstrated throughout your life. That's because you realized early on that you needed to act a certain way to protect yourself or ensure your survival. I've worked with many people whose relationships with their primary caregivers created a flawed and limited sense of self. In turn, this corrupted identity influenced the choices they made throughout their lives. Years of suffering and trauma have stemmed from the imprints of those early relationships.

This cannot be understated. The critical caregiver relationships or those people you looked to for validation in childhood have had a massive impact on your sense of value. They affected the magnitude of what you have believed possible for yourself and the size of the dreams you dreamed. They have also significantly influenced the actions you've taken or haven't taken throughout your life.

This can change.

In this moment you can see a new version of who you are that is free of any negative influence from your childhood. The effect of the nurturing of your past does not have to be a part of your future. What is interesting about any negative effect your nurturing had on your self-worth is that you can have a traumatic childhood and still have a drive for massive success and then achieve that success. Many throughout the world have demonstrated this fact. What this book focuses on, as a means to achieving a powerful mindset and attaining "success," is the mental power that emerges from realizing an inner sense of fulfillment, worth, and peace. Outer accomplishments without inner fulfillment or peace produce a hollow feeling. Many who run from an unsettled inner self keep chasing more material success or indulge in activities that produce a lot of adrenaline and short-term distraction. However, they find that they get no closer to ultimate freedom of mind this way. Self-mastery and an invincible mindset emerge through inner clarity and peace. Inner peace is a result of understanding the truth of who you are. This includes a new understanding of how you may have unknowingly and mistakenly, through no fault of your own, thought less of yourself due to a lack of nurturing or to trauma and physical or mental abuse from the caregivers and extremely influential people of your childhood.

THE IMPACT OF YOUR GENETICS: NATURE

The second element that has had a major impact on your identity is your genetics. Genetics are not just the carriers of hair color, face shape, skin color, and eye color. This coding is not just the determinant of health conditions and physical manifestations such as baldness or arthritis. Genetics endows us with hundreds of traits, instincts, and psychological behavior patterns from previous generations. There is a reason that as we age people often say to us, "Wow, you look and talk just like your father" or, "You have your mom's instincts, good taste, and laugh." The genes that were passed on to us at conception express different characteristics and instinctual tendencies that the previous generations used to survive. Surviving in this context can mean continuing to live or coping with life in a way that worked in a particular time and culture.

> **Genetics are a subtle and under-the-radar influence on your instincts, actions, and reactions.**

Genetic predispositions and inclinations toward certain behaviors and experiences can be positive or negative. They can promote optimism, joy, unlimited thinking, and a general fearlessness about life. Or they can carry past traumas, fears, sensitivities, phobias, predisposition to addiction, and other limiting beliefs and behaviors.

Think about your current personality. What dominant personality traits have you received from your mother? Which ones have you received from your father? Or rather, since these can be difficult to see in ourselves, which traits and attitudes have others told you match those of your parents or relatives in some way? Which traits from your parents or relatives have you purposely tried to avoid?

The reason I ask you to think about genetics (or the "nature" aspect of your identity) is that doing so helps you understand why you have had certain behavioral inclinations and responses over the years. Genetics may also explain why your general experience with relationships, money, or certain circumstances has followed a similar pattern to that of your parent or parents. Included in these patterns may be certain life choices that may have remained a complete mystery to you up until this point.

This understanding is not an excuse for or an acceptance of any past undesired actions. It is about gaining clarity regarding why you may have made those past choices. Regardless of this understanding, each person must still experience the consequences and karma of these past choices. The critical awareness you gain from realizing the influence of your genetics enables you to redirect these unwanted instincts and change them in the future.

One example of this is how children of the same parents

decide to interpret and respond to their parents' behavioral traits. If drinking alcohol was common in the household while growing up, one child may decide to summon the will to override any behavioral inclinations and never drink a drop of alcohol their entire life, while another child from the same household will find drinking to be a necessary and natural way of coping with everyday life.

Each person is born completely different, and each person gets a unique mix of genetic coding from both sides of their family tree. This is true even in the incredible case of identical twins. While the DNA at *conception* is a 100 percent match for identical twins, the genome of identical twins begins to change as they develop in the womb. At birth there is already a small percentage of genetic differences.

There have been endless studies of identical twins who have been separated at birth and reunited later in life. What researchers found is that the expression of their genes changed substantially throughout the years due to environmental influence. Studies like these are at the heart of environmental epigenetic research (the study of how environmental influences affect the expression of our genes) and offers a peek into how evolution works in real time.

The important takeaway is that you didn't choose the social, psychological, and physiological tendencies and inclinations that were passed on to you through your genes. This is a critical understanding in terms of personal forgiveness and peace. However, regardless of the genetic makeup you've been given or even how that genetic makeup has influenced your life up until this point, through awareness and intention, you can change these tendencies and patterns.

THE IMPACT OF YOUR PERSONAL EXPERIENCES: MEMORY

The third element that has significantly influenced your identity is your personal experiences. Since early childhood, you have had many meaningful experiences that have shaped your identity and how you see the world. Each experience, positive or negative, has influenced you and determined what you believed to be true. This has shaped your reality by way of an endless number of interpretations and reactions stemming from these core memories and adopted beliefs.

Here are some examples of how your personal experiences could have caused you to develop a negative, limited view of yourself, your potential, and your power. These experiences could have caused you to believe you are unworthy or even worthless in different ways:

"My dad, mom, caregivers, other family members, teachers, religious leaders, or friends _____."

- despised me
- ignored me
- physically abused me
- dismissed me

- laughed at and made fun of me
- controlled me
- made all my decisions for me
- lied to me
- sexually abused me
- abandoned me
- never heard me
- emotionally abused me
- manipulated me
- disapproved of me
- showed favor to others over me

These experiences at a young age may have had a major influence on how you valued yourself for years. As you will learn throughout this book, any self-deprecating thoughts are in opposition to the greater truth that life is showing you now and will continue to show you throughout the rest of your life.

The following examples of personal experiences could have caused you to develop an identity that has been dominated by fear or paranoia:

- You witnessed a tragedy where someone was seriously injured or died.
- Someone close to you died suddenly.
- A dog, cat, or other animal attacked you.
- You watched a lot of negative news programming.

- You watched a lot of negative or violent television shows or movies.
- You were shamed or exposed to negative or fear-based religious teachings.
- A person or a group at school bullied you.
- You were involved in a car accident.
- Someone bombarded you with fear and negativity about life.
- Someone attacked you.
- You were indoctrinated with negative and fear-dominated political rants.
- You were mentally, physically, or emotionally abused.
- You took a fall that caused injury.
- You had a sports injury.
- You had a traumatic swimming experience.

Any of these experiences could have traumatized you, causing you to believe that it's highly probable that something bad will happen to you in the future. These experiences and the resulting beliefs may have caused years of irrational fear and anxiety. This is the only truth about your future: anything is possible, and this includes millions of positive outcomes.

The following are examples of potential life experiences that could have created self-trust issues, doubts, or limiting beliefs about your ability to be successful in relationships, business, sports, or life in general:

- a traumatic breakup
- a business decision that caused a failure
- a key moment in sports when you did not perform well
- being fooled or conned out of money
- a time a client left you
- a low or failing grade on a test or in a class
- being cheated on in a relationship
- being suddenly fired
- being passed over for a promotion or a raise
- an investment decision you made that was unsuccessful
- a time you said something unbecoming or embarrassing that cost you in some way
- a time you were berated by a coach for not being successful

These experiences could have left you with a diminished view of what you are capable of or worthy of creating. Again, none of the resulting self-limiting beliefs are true.

An endless number of examples could be used to demonstrate how you have shaped your belief system about yourself and the world over the years. This process is especially impactful during the impressionable ages of six to thirteen. Interestingly, these personal experiences are connected to the nature (genetics) and nurturing you received that established your outlook on life and set your life in motion.

Some years ago, I discussed an example of the power of beliefs with a client. The conversation and the process of awareness were as follows:

ME: So tell me why these negative thoughts fill your head.

CLIENT: They just do. It's a constant voice in my head telling me what I can't do, what a failure I am, and how worthless I feel. It's been consistent since I was young. Probably from my absent dad and extremely negative mother.

ME: Do these thoughts help you?

CLIENT: Obviously not. Unless my goal is to continue to feel like shit every day.

ME: So, what is your goal?

CLIENT: I want this feeling to change! I want relief from this constant hopeless feeling.

ME: To do that, you have to start with seeing the truth about yourself.

CLIENT: What truth, that I screwed up my life so far?

ME: No, hardly. The truth that your past choices were based on the best understanding you had at that time.

CLIENT: Lovely, so I was stupid. I should have made different choices.

ME: No, you were not stupid. You were surviving the only way you knew how at the time. You reacted to your circumstances based on what you thought was your best option at that moment. Did you have perfect positive role models as parents, who had it all figured out? Were you shown the perfect choices to make and how to make them? Were you shown the best way to think and be as a child? Were you given any guidance on how to live an empowered life?

CLIENT: Ha, hardly. My mother was mentally ill and I don't

think my dad ever cared about me. Actually, I know he didn't because he left us. My mom used to beat me and tell me I was worthless and that I would never find anybody to marry almost every day. She pinned my nose at night with a clothespin to try and "thin it out" to make me look better. She was constantly yelling. She hated herself and was always trying to harm herself by trying to scratch her skin off. She tried to commit suicide three or four times after my father left us.

ME: So to blame yourself for any of the choices you've made in your life is completely unfair, unwarranted, and illogical. You've had some traumatic nurturing, and I'm sure your mother's nurturing as a child was no different. It may have been a dominant part of your family's genetic line. Basically, chaos seems to have been a big part of your family history, and because of that, it's permeated to a certain degree into the way you've seen and experienced yourself and your world. I'll say it again: you've done nothing wrong. You've survived the best way you knew how to this point. You're here now because you're tired of the way you've been surviving. You wouldn't be here if you didn't believe there was something different for you to experience. Let's keep working to change that experience. There is so much more for you to learn about yourself!

CLIENT: Jeez, it feels so weird to look back without feeling bad. I guess I didn't realize how much this rampant negativity has been there my entire life. It's felt so common.

Chaos and negativity were just a part of my everyday childhood.

ME: Exactly. You didn't know the difference, so how could you possibly do any different? Also, if this new perspective feels different, we are on the right path. Truth can feel this way at first. It's a good thing.

CLIENT: It feels very weird but very relieving, actually.

Remember, none of the degrading or self-limiting conclusions you've drawn from any of the traumatic experiences of your past are true. They are false beliefs and limit your true, infinite potential.

You may have had many unfortunate experiences, but these events have nothing to do with the probability of what *will* happen unless you continue to put the energy of your attention on them. The only true thing is that in this moment you are capable of creating anything you can conceive of, believe in, and work toward. (If you don't believe this yet, I encourage you to return to step one.)

STAY PRESENT IN THE SPACE OF INFINITE POSSIBILITY

There is a very important part of your psyche that is in charge of your reality. Your ego is the mental mechanism that bridges your beliefs to your experience. It is also designed to protect you and defend these beliefs. Memory is one way it accomplishes this protection. If a person hurt you in your past, your ego will be on high alert for any similar conditions that may cause this hurt again. The ego will look for patterns to prevent you from suffering again. It will cause you to be cautious of putting yourself in similar situations that may cause pain. In other words, depending on the previous pain and suffering, the ego will trigger you to be cautious, distrustful, or guarded. This makes sense in certain circumstances as we are all required to learn and adjust so we don't get hurt again. However, the poison in the well appears when you project negative outcomes on your future or feel unworthy in any way due to past difficult experiences.

The following two truths immediately dissolve any future negative projections:

1. Every moment of life is distinct and unique.

2. In each moment, there are infinite possibilities available to us for creation.

The most successful people in the world operate from a mindset that looks for the valuable information in any negative or unsuccessful experience. Failure motivates them. They learn from it and then move forward in the next moment with a strong belief in a positive outcome. They do not put a negative bias on a future that hasn't happened yet. They do not let any previous experience or person affect what they believe is possible for themselves. They use all experiences as information to help them get closer to achieving their creative intention. Great athletes are perfect examples of this process of perseverance.

Eternal optimism about yourself and life is a key to being a powerful, conscious creator.

No matter what has happened in your life, liberating yourself from any limiting thoughts that impede the infinite possibilities available to you now will help you achieve an invincible state of mind. Understanding how the driving creative force of your life, your identity, has come together is a big step in the journey to a higher state of awareness, and ultimately the mindset of infinite potential and personal liberation. You've done the best you can up to this point with what you've known and with the teachings and nurturing that have embedded in your mind since birth. There is no value in holding any regrets. Conversely, there is freedom of mind and empowerment in understanding the reasons for so many of your past choices and actions. It's time to take more conscious control of the process!

STEP 2 REFLECTION QUESTIONS

Answer the following reflection questions to determine if you're ready to move on to step three. If you can't confidently answer every question with yes, write down why you currently feel this way. Keep your responses with those from the end of step one.

1. Do you realize that your past is the result of a creative process you had not been fully aware of?

2. Do you understand why gaining awareness about your past is critical to what you desire?

3. Do you realize the impact your nurturing and upbringing have had on your identity, beliefs, and way of looking at the world?

4. Do you realize how your genetics and the experiences of your ancestors have influenced your personality and your life up to this moment?

5. Do you realize how your personal experiences have shaped your identity, beliefs, and view of yourself and the world?

6. Do you realize that any negative or limiting thoughts about your identity are false?

7. Do you know you did the best you could have up to this point based on how your identity has come together?

DIRECTING YOUR EGO

How to Consciously Create Your Present and Positively Shape Your Future

The future depends on what you do today.
—Mahatma Gandhi

Just as it is critical to understand the way your identity was formed and shaped throughout your past, it is important for you to realize how your identity is related to what you are creating now. Your current perceptions and thoughts determine what's probable for you to create for your future. This process is driven by the mechanism within you that is designed to protect, defend, create, and validate your truth: your ego. Becoming acutely aware of how your ego operates through your thoughts and actions is how you consciously create the life you desire.

Let's use a real-time example. You have absorbed the words

in front of you because of your intention to understand more about how life works. Through an endless number of beautiful synchronicities, this book made its way into your hands, magnetized by you and your intention to know. This book is just one piece of an endless stream of resources available to you. This example reveals the co-creative relationship between you and life. Life is unconditionally here to help you manifest your intentions. You always have a choice regarding how much you decide to implement the information that shows up in your life. That is your free will. It is these moment-by-moment decisions that determine your evolving destiny.

THE IMPACT OF YOUR BELIEFS

Your identity has influenced all your perceptions, actions, and reactions, and hence your experiences of your past. The constitution of your identity *right now* will determine your perceptions, actions, and reactions in this moment and thus determine many of your future experiences. The important takeaway is that what you believe about who you are right now determines not only exactly what your ego will seek to experience but also how life will prepare to meet you in the coming moments.

Your life can't change until there is a fundamental shift in your identity and view of life. Why? Because life, your co-creative partner in this process, can only serve your core truths, for better or for worse. A major part of demonstrating a mindset of infinite potential is becoming aware of how life connects to your beliefs and leads to the creation of your reality.

To life, it's all creative. Positive or negative is irrelevant. Life is simply looking to mirror your dominant beliefs. Understanding this process to its core is life-changing. You cannot change your life or achieve new results when you don't know what to change. You can't change your life when you aren't ready for the change. And you certainly aren't going to create new results when you deny or avoid what needs to be changed. Have you ever tried to offer someone the truth that would help change their life when they weren't ready to hear it? It's not a fun process. When it comes to looking at the truth, readiness is everything!

Life works with you and supports you in two major ways:

- by magnetizing the conditions around you to match or create what you believe is true
- by working to shatter any ignorance you have about what is true *in relation to* what you desire to experience

This process is exact.

THE JOB OF YOUR EGO

How you define yourself through the beliefs that start with "I AM" is what your ego looks to validate and protect as real.

Seeking the validation of who you believe you are becomes the ego's job. This process is how you feel alive and know you exist. You can dream of love or think you're loved, but your soul eventually wants to feel or experience love. You can imagine being a great athlete or think you are a great one, but your soul ultimately wants to experience this by working toward it physically and hopefully achieving this goal. You can imagine being successful at your job or think you are a success, but your soul wants to feel success through an experience of a successful result at work. When your mind is not convinced that a specific part of your identity is being validated, it puts the ego in active mode to accomplish this.

The mechanism or bridge that takes your intention and moves it to an experience is the ego. Your ego only follows the instructions from your truth. Your truth drives your intentions. Your ego does not care if your truth is negative or positive. *This is why it is so critical to be self-aware and know what you really think of yourself.* If you feel you are stupid or an embarrassment ("I AM stupid"), your ego will look to create experiences or emotions that validate this self-limiting idea. An example would be blurting out an inappropriate comment that you immediately regret in a conversation with a coworker, giving you the feeling of being stupid. You may wonder what compelled you to say such a thing, yet it is an example of the ego subconsciously accomplishing its goal of validating a negative belief.

If you have a fear of failure ("I AM a failure"), your ego will work hard to prove this to you by focusing on an experience that makes you feel like a failure. An example would be continuing to beat yourself up over a poor athletic performance or a bad financial decision that caused a loss of money.

If you feel you are not worthy of finding a lasting loving relationship ("I AM unworthy of love"), life will put together the conditions that lead your ego to validate this negative truth. You may continue to choose relationships in which you are lied to, cheated on, or manipulated in ways that bring you to the circumstance that "proves" that these negative feelings or fears are true. This creative process is a demonstration of a self-fulfilling prophecy.

Any time you are not at peace with who you believe you are, your ego will go to work to reconcile the imbalance of mind.

How hard your ego works or the level of panic you feel is based on how intolerable the current circumstance is to you. In addition, the more a particular belief you have about yourself or your life reflects your ignorance, the more life will meet you with the conditions that either keep you in conflict with reality because of the ignorance or provide a circumstance that shatters the false belief.

Why will life sometimes shatter a personal truth? Because life is connecting to you based on your intentions. Life serves your intentions by increasing the probability that they manifest. If you are ignorant about something that prevents you from accomplishing your intent, life must reveal this ignorance to you. It will use the path of least resistance to accomplish this task. Shattering a false belief is one way it will accomplish this. For people who are very stubborn, think they are never wrong, or are very resistant to change, this can be a very painful process.

Here are some common examples of what I call *ignorance-shattering experiences*:

- You think you can handle a high speed and you lose control of your car and get in a bad accident.
- You think your significant other will never leave you no matter how you treat them, and one day you walk into an empty home.
- You think you are stupid until a good, caring teacher tells you how valuable you are and how much potential is in you for greatness.
- You think your stock or real estate investment can't go down in value, and suddenly you're selling the investment at a massive loss.
- You think you are incapable of getting sick and are stronger than any virus, and then you're down for the count.
- You think the world is just a cold dark place until you randomly experience the love and kindness of a stranger.
- You think you can handle your addiction, until your life turns to chaos because of its impact on your health, relationships, job, or financial situation.

- You think life doesn't support you, until you realize that life is guiding you right now.

THE PURPOSE OF KARMA

Whenever you are ignorant of any truth about yourself or life, you create karma. The karma is that you will eventually have to experience a lesson of awareness. How that lesson shows up is the interesting part. The degree of suffering that accompanies the karma is correlated to the degree of ignorance and stubbornness of the person. I once heard, "As with egos and trees, the bigger they are, the harder they fall."

Any illusions you have about life and how it works are destined to be revealed as false along your evolutionary journey. It's only a matter of when. Everyone is headed toward truth. The simple reason is that truth is a necessary component of evolution and survival.

Your beliefs have worked to shape your perception of life. Once your beliefs were set, and for most of your adult life, you worked to see what you wanted to see and hear what you wanted to hear each day to make sure your view of yourself and the world stayed intact. There have been many startling disruptions to this view along the way as life has shown you its evolving truth.

There are many examples of large disruptions. The COVID-19 pandemic demonstrated that some emerging viruses are more damaging and life-threatening than others. The 9/11 terrorist attacks in Washington, DC, and New York City demonstrated that the United States is more vulnerable to sabotage than we once thought. Another instance might be the day you found out that Santa Claus isn't real. Or the time you were presented with news and factual data on global warming that demonstrated that our earth's climate is changing and has environmental and economic consequences.

Each of these events has affected your worldview and your current identity differently. Some of these startling and often-disappointing truths you have accepted, and some you have resisted. For people who are insecure or fearful, any facts or truths that dissolve what their ego wants to protect as real (or that may puncture a "bubble of delusion") are deemed irrelevant, rationalized, attacked, or avoided altogether. For people who have experienced a lot of trauma in their lives or who have big issues with trust and vulnerability, alternate theories are an easy way to validate a manipulative or oppressive worldview, make sense of any unknown circumstances, and avoid real truths. When self-described "fair and trusted" media sources put out false and fear-based information about important and emotional issues, they can snare millions of people into this trap. Once your mind is caught in this sort of fear trap, your fear is like a fishhook that sets. It's even harder to pull back and free yourself because this would mean admitting you were manipulated or conned. Hence this maxim from Mark Twain: "It's easier to fool people than to convince them that they have been fooled."

When you live in a dominant state of fear or insecurity, you are less likely to have an open mind and self-reflect. Your ego shuts off self-reflection and the ability to learn. Why? Because your ego must protect the belief that your fears, insecurities, or mistrust of the world are real in order to hold your known identity together. The massive danger in this way of living is that you cut yourself off from insight, knowledge, truth, and conscious growth. You limit the beautiful ability in you to exhibit discernment and evolve. Everything your ego does becomes about protecting your worldview and about being "right." Objectivity is completely lost. This is all in an effort to avoid accepting any disruptive truths or to avoid feelings of guilt, shame, and regret for being wrong or feeling like you got conned. The problem with this type of self-protection is that you end up being stuck in time and in a state of perpetual suffering due to your rejection of truth, your unwillingness to adapt, or your general paranoid and negative outlook. Ironically, this resistance starts to confirm your fears as you slowly destroy your life in this close-minded, imbalanced state. Only the truth can set you free.

The inability to self-reflect and admit when you're incorrect is the path to suffering.

The happiest people in the world are the most positive, optimistic, humble, self-reflecting, and self-aware. They have the ability to open up and embrace truth and flow with change. Self-awareness prevents the resistance that can cause anger and other self-preserving emotions in response to new life-changing information in the world. Resistance to truth keeps you in a state of delusion and ignorance and takes you down a road of self-destruction and chaos. Self-reflection and a mind open to truth, on the other hand, allow you to see how a new understanding of the situation may align with better choices and more peaceful and successful outcomes for your life.

Remember, any past ignorance and the unfortunate suffering it caused do not make you any less worthy of ultimately having what you desire. It is absolutely your responsibility to acknowledge the past, learn, and change, but you are not in any way unworthy because of your past.

Delusion is the result of years and sometimes lifetimes of misaligned beliefs and negative experiences. It is the combination of fears and memories of pain and trauma. Your ego was just protecting you from the fear of more suffering or the fear of feeling bad again because you had to admit or accept that you were incorrect. Instead, your ego may have done the opposite, costing you more time and suffering because of your resistance. The key to living more powerfully and mentally free is to accept truth as factually presented and learn as fast as you can. To not be afraid of being "wrong" but to be more excited about what you can learn that is "right." You have done the best you could have up to this moment. If you could have done better in the past with any of your choices or decisions, you would have. All that matters is what you want to experience from this moment forward. Greater objectivity and openness of mind put you in the most optimal state of creation.

YOUR EGO IS YOUR ALLY

Contrary to popular belief, you can control your ego. The invincible mindset entails becoming more conscious of the ego's process, so you know exactly what commands you are giving your ego and what perceptions, actions, and reactions you want to exhibit to define who you choose to be and create a new result.

Your ego dictates the quality of the energy of all your thoughts and feelings. Every minute of every day, your ego is working to either create or destroy based only on what will validate your truth. In a way, the term *ego* can be looked at as an acronym for the phrase "energy goes out."

Your ego is your biggest ally, protector, and friend. It is what is navigating and captaining your experience of life. It is *not* something to be controlled or destroyed. It is simply waiting to be directed. It is the regulator of your state of mind. Every single person has an ego.

THE PASSIVE EGO AND THE ACTIVE EGO

There are two modes of your ego that determine your daily energy. There is the *passive ego*, which is simply operating the daily tasks that define who you are—for example, getting up at a certain time, taking a shower, driving to work, going to the grocery store, or engaging in a friendly way with people. And there is the *active ego*, which engages when there is a threat to one of your beliefs in some way. When the active ego is engaged, reality is not validating what you believe is true, someone is challenging who you are, or you are simply insecure about what you believe is true and are trying to compensate in some way through the expression of your energy. The more out of touch a person is with reality, the more their ego will be working to reconcile that discrepancy. When an ego is constantly in an active state, it's known as either a "big ego" or an "unstable ego." People with these types of egos (unconsciously) work hard to convince themselves and the world that they are not what their negative voice tells them they are.

This behavior could manifest as boasting or constantly flaunting expensive possessions such as jewelry and cars, or always insisting that one knows everything or is always right. It could show up as drug use, thrill seeking, drinking, sexual promiscuity, gambling, or attachment to extreme political parties, gangs, or cults. Basically, these actions include anything people can do to distract themselves or make themselves feel better because they feel internally unstable. The problem occurs when the negative feeling doesn't go away on the inside no matter how much one tries to compensate for it on the outside. Attempting to feel good about yourself by focusing only on external possessions or thrill-seeking actions is like trying to put your fingers in several leaks in a dam that you're afraid might break—the leaks will keep coming and you don't have enough fingers to plug every hole. Without dealing with the source of the leaks, it's an exhausting way to live.

People with big or unstable egos are really struggling internally to find peace and self-worth. They feel valueless and doubtful and are trying desperately to compensate for those feelings. A person with a big or active ego simply needs more validation that they are who they "think" they are than someone with a small ego does.

Conversely, the person with a passive or small ego is more content and secure with who they are. Therefore, the ego doesn't need to do as much protecting and validating. Who they "think" and experience they are is more in line with who they know they are. The ego is less noticeable in these individuals, and in some cases the person may even seem to have "no ego" or be "egoless."

It's no wonder that those who practice Buddhism work to rid themselves of attachments and outer identity. They shave their heads, take new names, and wear same-colored robes. It's a radical approach of countering a needy ego by reducing any outer symbolism related to the individual self. People who practice Buddhism adopt these practices to help free the mind; reveal the unattached, limitless self; reduce suffering; and know peace.

THE TRUTH ABOUT CHASING PERFECTION

An active ego can also manifest as "perfectionism." This is not to be confused with individuals who are looking to be great at what they do and reach higher levels of performance.

What I'm referring to here are individuals who feel so unworthy on the inside that they search for perfection in everything they do and are highly critical of themselves and others. Because perfection is so hard to attain, they rarely feel good enough, so it's a constant chase with little joy. For these individuals a feeling of being perfect rarely comes and never lasts.

This reminds me of a comment from a thirteen-year-old boy I was working with. His father had divorced his mother and completely abandoned him. He looked up to his father and had idolized him in every way. His father had gone on to marry someone else, had started a new family, and wasn't giving the young teen the time of day. As a result, the teen felt anxious, depressed, and worthless. To attempt to solve the issue, he became an absolute perfectionist. He thought that if he demonstrated perfection, he would gain his father's love and attention again. If not that, at least he would protect himself from ever being abandoned again. His thought was, *Who would want to discard someone who is perfect?* He became obsessed with being perfect at everything. One comment he made really stood out to me. He was talking about how he performed on the tests he took at school, and he said, "Even when I get a perfect score on a test, I stress and wonder if the teacher asked the perfect questions." Until this teenager realized the truth of his perfection, with or without his father's love, no data or feedback demonstrating his perfection would convince him of this truth.

You cannot run from who you are. Who you are is defined by what you believe about yourself. But you can change what you believe and hence change who you are.

A feeling of unworthiness is not a tolerable state of mind. The ego actively avoids this feeling at all costs. As a result, avoidance of the truth, creation of false narratives about reality, relief of the mind through drug use, and other destructive and desperate survival actions will emerge. The ego simply scrambles for constant validation or a method to feel better when experiencing the pain of feeling unworthy. The conundrum is that, just as a dog chasing its tail will never catch it, a person who does not change the false belief of "I don't matter" will never achieve peace in the soul through any outer change in their reality.

That is why the ultimate path to empowerment is self-understanding and awareness. Awareness lifts your soul with the truth of the worthiness of who you are and the realization of the infinite possibilities of who you can become. It makes you impenetrable to any of the negativity in your universe. When you are self-aware, no one or no "thing" can manipulate you or throw you off-balance. You are centered in self-understanding, and therefore your ego is ready for anything and, in turn, can shield you from any negativity. When you are not grounded in self-understanding, you become susceptible to suffering. Your ego can create negative ideas and experiences that keep you from attaining peace of mind and making your dreams a reality.

WHAT THE EGO REVEALS ABOUT YOUR BELIEFS

Evaluating your ego's actions and reactions can be a very quick and powerful way to see where there has been an insecurity in your belief system or a conflict with truth.

For example, say a family member says you're not a caring individual. If their opinion matters to you, your ego will go into red alert, an active protection mode. This is because their harsh words are invalidating a part of what defines who you are. This may cause your blood pressure to rise and may move your ego into a hyper-defensive mode to protect your character.

Keep in mind that in some instances harsh words from another may need your attention because they actually convey a certain truth. This is why you always have to be honest with yourself about your behavior. In other cases, harsh words are simply the other person's form of mental and emotional manipulation. Such behavior may have gone on for years. If this manipulation has been a common experience, you can start to change it.

Your ego's reaction gives you clues about what you need. In the case of the family member who says you're not caring, you need that person to see you as a caring individual. If you know you've been a caring individual and you've made that clear, then the immediate way to take back control of your state of mind is to drop the *need* to prove anything to them. Keep being who you want to be, but do not allow them to manipulate you and your emotions through your need for their approval. If you know you've been caring, there is no need for any outside validation. After you take back your power by dropping the need for their approval and validation, any further comments of theirs won't affect your identity. This is because your identity is no longer predicated on their opinion. Your ego will have no reaction (and will be in a passive mode), so you will stay in emotional balance. True self-mastery is taking complete control over what affects your state of mind.

Be warned: others may get even more upset at your non-reaction to their manipulation. Your path, if you want to be in the most productive mindset, is to stay in your truth no matter what they say or do to try to throw you off-balance. It is a matter of will. How badly do you want to stay in a peaceful state of mind? The more you need others' approval, the more power you give them to manipulate your precious state of mind.

Consider an example about romantic relationships: if the belief "I AM unworthy of love" is deeply embedded in your identity, your ego will look to prove this unworthiness to you in every romantic relationship you create. It will find reasons to work toward the end of a relationship rather than fostering a deeper connection. If vulnerability caused pain at some point in your childhood or adult life and your ego linked pain to vulnerability, then your ego will not allow you to be vulnerable in relationships. The ego must validate what you believe to be true about yourself. This will go on until you change the sponsoring false belief about yourself or your life.

Say you're an athlete who's worried about your future performance because of the embedded belief "I AM not good enough." You anxiously ask yourself, "Will I play? Will I play well? Will the coach start me? Will I get a scholarship? Will I go pro?" This reaction is caused by the ego's desperate need for a sense of certainty that these things will happen, but the concern is being supported by a destructive belief. The ego's response reveals that you are both uncertain of what you will accomplish and in need of validation that you will accomplish it. This distracts you from your power and puts your mind on a negative outcome. In this scenario, there is a lack of faith. The only thing your mind *should* be focused on for the best performance is what you *can* control. Factors like your preparation and your focus when you play. And most importantly, your belief in yourself. This is what brings results, and results are what takes care of every question the nervous ego is asking. Even more importantly, results end the questioning. To move in this more productive and positive direction, you need to first change your core beliefs.

CLIENT: Why am I so fearful of putting myself out there?

ME: You have pain from a past experience and an ego that's telling you you'll experience pain in your future if you try again.

CLIENT: Will I?

ME: It's impossible to know the future. The ego has no clue, regardless of what it's trying to tell you. Only you can make that determination. The key is to be willing to try either way, knowing you'll be OK regardless.

CLIENT: I am telling you I am fearful!

ME: And so it is ...

CLIENT: What?!

ME: You're making a negative declaration about continuing to be fearful. A powerful one that starts with "I AM." What do you think your ego is going to do? Allow you to go through with trying again? Not a chance. If you want to *not* feel as fearful, then you have to see that fear is not helping you get any closer to what you really want. You have to adopt a different state of mind and attitude about what you are doing and send your ego new instructions. You have to trust the process and know that moving forward with faith and courage is the way, no matter what the short-term outcome is. It is this faith and a new belief about your worth that will reduce your fear.

CLIENT: So I have to trust that I'll be OK?

ME: Yes! Exactly! If you want to move forward and enjoy a new experience, you must summon the will to move forward no matter what. There are millions of possibilities for you to experience, including endless positive ones. You have to send new instructions to your ego about what you believe is possible and who you believe you are. Your will to experience what you know in the deepest part of you is possible has to be stronger than any negative projection. There is no other way to achieve what you want.

CLIENT: So telling my ego I'm afraid right now is making me feel afraid and stopping me from moving forward?

ME: Exactly. It's honoring your truth. How about if you instead took on the mindset that you're excited? Excited to try, to learn, to conquer, and to advance in any way with the opportunity in front of you! What if you adopted the belief that nothing could hurt you? If you do this, your whole mindset will shift and you will focus on moving forward with a positive attitude. What if you decided to look at every experience as if it were working for you? Then nothing could stop you!

CLIENT: Well, that would definitely be different.

ME: How exciting is that to know? If you have gotten this far with a mindset and ego that have been negative and working against you and what you want at times, imagine what you could do and accomplish with a mind and ego that are working toward your desires!

CLIENT: Wow, yeah, that's cool . . . But why would my ego work against my desires?

ME: Because the ego doesn't care about your desires. It only cares about your truth. If your truth is "I can't" or "I'm fearful" or "I'll get hurt," the ego will make sure you experience that. It has to validate what you believe is true about you. But that's what's so exciting! Take the vital time necessary to work to change your truth, which you're doing right now, and watch the magic that happens!

HOW YOUR TRUTH GOVERNS YOUR EGO

The bottom line is that no matter what you want or intend to experience, your truth will have the final say on what happens. The ego has no choice. This can occur in a destructive (negative) way or a creative (positive) way. During this process, life continues to provide you with the lessons that move you toward more of the expansive truth of who you really are. This is not a path of destruction but rather a path of beautiful creation.

Here is a powerful thing to remember regarding how to take control and manage your ego when you feel you are starting to get in an emotionally charged state. If something happens during your day that creates a conflict in your mind or someone tries to provoke you with a negative comment, stop, take a breath, and ask yourself this very powerful question:

Who do I choose to be now?

The answer to this question will immediately send instructions to your ego, which in turn will determine the exact energy and response that aligns with this answer. This is a way to stay more consciously on top of pivotal moments of your day that you want to change so they are more in line with who you desire to be. *This is how you take control over how the probabilities for your future experiences unfold.* Consciously directing your ego in the manner you desire is pivotal to changing your future for the better. A mind that is more in harmony with your soul's true desire results in an ego that is more re-laxed and serendipitously working to elevate your entire life.

When your mind is calm and you have a solid under-standing of who you are, your ego is more passive. This is like having the best captain and crew on your boat. You have mapped out a plan; you take the shortest, safest route; and you use the winds and currents to your advantage for speed and to save precious time. When a person is grounded in ac-ceptance and confidence in who they are, they exhibit a calm-ness and a Zen-like energy. They experience very smooth sailing through life, even through the ups and downs and any unavoidable storms or moments of change. Serendipity becomes commonplace.

When you see how fast manifestation occurs when you align your dreams with the truth of who you really are, you will understand your true power in life.

Now that you know how your ego works to manage your experience of reality and how your awareness of this positively influences your future, you are ready to discover the self-limiting beliefs that have been the obstacles preventing you from achieving more of what is possible for you. Removing these limits will allow you to fully express your soul and break through to the reality and results you really desire. Once these obstacles of mind have been revealed, they can be dissolved!

STEP 3 REFLECTION QUESTIONS

Answer yes or no to the following reflection questions to determine if you're ready to move on to step four. If you answer any of the questions with no, write down why you currently feel this way. Keep your responses with those from the preceding steps.

1. Do you realize that your truth ("I AM...") can be different from what you think you believe about yourself?

2. Do you realize that your ego's job is to validate your truth whether it's negative or positive, conscious or subconscious, in line with your desires or not?

3. Do you realize that life is always helping you create what you desire or working to show you where you are ignorant of the truth that will help you create?

4. Do you realize that your ego is a protector, defender, and ally of your identity?

5. Do you realize that an active ego reveals where you are not in harmony with the truth?

6. Do you know that you can change the way your ego works so that it seeks to construct your life in favor of what you desire?

DISMANTLING
SELF-LIMITING BELIEFS

How to Free Your Mind

Man stands in his own shadow and wonders
why it's dark.

—Zen proverb

In step three, you learned how your state of mind and the
way you define who you are determine what you create in
this moment and the probabilities for what you will create
in the future. This process reveals how much power you hold
in every moment.

Inspired by this knowledge, you might ask the next logical question: "What is preventing me or limiting me from
moving toward more of what I want to experience?" Or, if you
have been moving toward your goal or vision, the appropriate

question may be, "What beliefs have been preventing my goals from manifesting, and what has kept me from breaking through to the next level of results?" There are many people in the world whom I have seen manifest effortlessly. What is their secret? Step four will help you answer all these questions.

As you learned so far, life works to enlighten you, exposing any ignorance that has kept you from what you truly want. Therefore, to move the needle of probability in favor of your dreams materializing, you must examine your thoughts and beliefs through honest self-reflection to see which beliefs have been holding you back. These are called *limiting beliefs*. These are any thoughts you hold that say you are unworthy or incapable or any beliefs that limit a fuller expression of who you are.

THE POWER OF OVERCOMING LIMITING THOUGHTS

When moving in the direction of your dreams, you must be candid with yourself about what actions you're taking to increase the odds that your desired reality will emerge. You must be grounded in the understanding of what it takes in the particular system or field you are trying to work in to create what you desire. You have to be aware of the path to success in your arena and how to navigate it smartly.

It doesn't matter what your intent is; limiting beliefs, whether conscious or subconscious, will restrict your power to manifest what you want. Finding these mental limitations is a critical part of the process of dismantling these beliefs on the path to breaking through to new results. Once you can identify these false and counterproductive beliefs, you can challenge them. Once you challenge them, you finally have the real opportunity to change them.

In this step you will gain insight on how to reflect and find these limits and how to de-energize and dissolve them. A new idea of who you are will surface. With an authentic shift in how you look at yourself, you can authentically conceive a new reality. New results will follow.

The following example shows how a professional athlete changed his beliefs about what was possible for him and how this led to an incredible shift in his results. In 2014, Canadian professional golfer Nick Taylor was in his rookie season on the PGA Tour. He didn't have to wait long for his first victory. In only his fourth event as a PGA Tour professional, he won the Sanderson Farms Championship by two shots. The stage was set for a fast start to his career. Or at least that's what Nick thought.

Nick qualified for the PGA Tour in 2014, after a stellar amateur career playing for the University of Washington that included the Canadian amateur championship, the Ben Hogan Award for the best college player in the United States, and the rank of top amateur golfer in the world. Success was simply hardwired into his mind. There was no reason to think it wouldn't continue. However, three years later, in early 2017, he had not notched another victory.

Getting his first win so early in his career was both good

and bad. Good for the immediate validation and confidence it gave him. Bad for the very high expectations it set in his mind for what he "should" be accomplishing on the world's toughest stage. By 2017 Nick was in a situation where many weeks he was struggling just to make the cut to play the weekend and earn money. He was starting to become concerned not just about winning but about simply being more consistent, keeping his playing privileges on tour, and supporting his family. Now, three years since his first and only win, the situation was starting to get to him. However, as a relentless and determined competitor, he also knew it was time to look deeper for answers.

We started mental strength work together in early 2017. Immediately we found that over the last three years doubt had slowly crept in about what Nick believed was possible. In each tournament that didn't go well for him, more frustration, doubt, and angst crept into his mind. When you don't get results in life, you often start letting your mind slip into thinking about what is not possible rather than the truth of what is possible. This is especially true when your expectations become high. Then disappointment increases and limiting beliefs start creeping deep into the subconscious and start to negatively affect results. It happens in relationships after a bad breakup or two. It happens in business when you have a bad experience with a job. It is no different in sports. The difference with those who master their minds and achieve their dreams is that they stay open to possibility, they stay open to learning, and they keep going no matter what.

Those with an invincible mindset are unafraid to look at areas they need to improve to have better results, and they are unafraid to try new things. When they get knocked down, they have the will and resiliency to get back up and try again and again. They ignore any negative or limiting thoughts by staying focused only on what they believe is possible.

Nick has great resiliency, so the first thing we worked on was focusing his mind on all the possibilities that were in front of him each time he entered a tournament. We worked on conditioning his mind for less doubt and hence more faith in the process. We focused on turning around his internal energy through renewed optimism and hope. Armed with a new and more positive mental outlook on the possibilities and backed by his relentless physical and technical work on his game, Nick immediately saw a change in his results. Sometimes all it takes to spark a turnaround is a new attitude buoyed by a reminder of some inspirational truth. The truth Nick needed to hear was that nothing had ever stopped him from achieving all he already had achieved at every level of golf prior to this one. While tolerance for error and having a very sound strategy is certainly much tighter at the professional level, the process of competing and winning is no different. What is different is that at the professional level there are no weak intentions and mindsets among those who win or compete to win each week. These are the best players in the world. But there was no reason why Nick couldn't refresh his mind and attitude about himself and match that high level of intention and belief with his own.

Nick's confidence increased with each improved tournament result, as many of the limiting beliefs that had crept in over the past three years were *challenged and removed*. A major key was changing his mindset from a state of worry or a fixation on results to a focus on execution in the moment and optimism about his capabilities and level of talent. Another critical aspect of his mindset shift was reducing any negative emotion or resistance to imperfect shots, which can be counterproductive to decision making and better execution. While perfection is the aim, expecting it was getting in the way of creating it. Also, dismantling Nick's limiting belief that he had to hit the golf ball as far as some of the longer hitters on tour completely changed his energy.

In golf there are many styles of play and many ways to win. Being a very long driver of the golf ball is helpful but not imperative for winning. Great putting, a sharp short game, and—probably most important but least talked about—an incredibly smart strategy and mental approach are what truly separates the best from the rest. Nick applied all of these abilities.

In early 2020 Nick found himself at the AT&T Pebble Beach Pro-Am with a one-shot lead on the final day in the final group with five-time champion of the event and Hall of Famer Phil Mickelson. Not one of the expert analysts on the Golf Channel that morning picked Nick to win, even though he had the lead. Every single one picked Mickelson or major champion Jason Day, who was three shots back.

Nick and I anticipated that the big crowd would be pulling for Mickelson, and we prepared for it. This is when Phil

Mickelson was still on the tour and remained very popular. We also anticipated the crazy ways Mickelson would rally and make par or birdie during the round. Nick was quietly prepared for it all and ready to stay focused no matter what occurred. The plan was to play his game and have confidence in his strength. To trust himself and his incredible ball striking and competitive energy. The mental game plan was to not let a single doubt or limiting belief about what was possible enter his mind.

On a very windy day in Monterey, California, Nick Taylor started out hot, birdieing holes four and five and making an eagle at hole six to start four under par. Meanwhile, Mickelson was cold, starting out five over par after his first eight holes. Mickelson finally settled in and made three birdies on the back nine with the crowd clearly favoring him and cheering him on. Nick, however, stayed undeterred, and after a tough double bogey on the fourteenth hole, he bounced back, stayed completely locked in, and essentially closed out the victory with a beautiful chip in birdie to shock Mickelson on fifteen. He made one more birdie for good measure on the iconic seventeenth hole. He then walked up the beautiful eighteenth hole at Pebble Beach, his favorite golf course in the world, with a four-shot lead and a victory that would validate him with his second PGA Tour championship.

With that victory in the bag, we completely expanded the intentions for the rest of Nick's year and career. New goals were set to dismantle any old limits and to push his mind to completely new territory. Included on his goal list for 2020, 2021, and 2022 were contending in and winning more tournaments; winning his nation's biggest tournament, the Canadian Open; making the top fifty in the world rankings; and qualifying for the Olympics.

As his self-directed fate would have it, a little over a year after this goal work, at the Canadian Open in June 2023, Nick went into a playoff with Tommy Fleetwood of England, one of the top players in the world. On the fourth playoff hole, Nick sank what is now known in Canada as "the putt." He made a seventy-two-foot-long putt for birdie to become the first Canadian in sixty-nine years to win the Canadian Open. It was an incredible sports moment, especially for the country of Canada—check. In February 2024 Nick Taylor, with relentless focus and determination, birdied four of his last five holes to defeat seasoned professional Charley Hoffman in a playoff at the Phoenix Open to win the tournament—check. Nick moved up to be a top-thirty-ranked player in the world—check. In June 2023 Nick was selected as one of two Olympians to represent Canada at the 2024 Olympics in Paris—check. With a mind that is free from so many of his previous doubts and hidden limits, Nick has accomplished many of the goals he's been working on for years and is on his way to more.

Was this an overnight success? Absolutely not. Nick worked hard for many years to develop his talent. He had the ability and humility to continually face what wasn't working and to seek any information that would make him better. He did this consistently until it all came together for another significant breakthrough in performance and class. He trusted the process and refused to let his mind stop him from what he knew in his heart he was capable of creating. He then took the time to consecrate his goals by putting them on paper. He did all of this and had the critical vulnerability to work on his mindset to clear out any subconscious limits that were affecting his performance. He was willing to stretch his mind to overcome doubt and embrace new possibilities.

This same ability lies in *you*. Clearing your mind of any false beliefs that prevent you from embracing the most productive creative energy is a big part of achieving new breakthroughs and success. It also fosters a state of mind that streamlines the path to your deepest goals and desires. You must be ready to withstand every test that life deems necessary in order to build the invincible state of mind and create the conditions that lead to new levels of success.

LEARNING THROUGH ACTION AND FAITH

When a farmer has the intention to plant and harvest a crop, they must know exactly what seed they want to plant. The farmer must make sure the seed is of high quality and will produce a good crop. They must prepare the soil to make it fertile for planting. They must water the field. And once the conditions are in place, the farmer must have the patience and faith to let life work its creative magic as the seed germinates and grows. When the crop emerges from the soil, the farmer must nurture and protect it. Consistently watering and guarding it from predators must be part of the process to make sure the crop grows strong. The farmer cannot rush to harvest the crop too early, or it won't be ripe. There is a timing to the process and a keen awareness of the proper nurturing along the way to the desired end result. If the farmer takes their eye off the crop, it may not get enough water, it may be eaten by animals, or the soil might become depleted of nutrients. This lack of awareness will delay the success of the farmer's crop or ruin it altogether. Also, the seed has to be strong, because if the seed is weak, no matter how much work and nurturing the farmer does, the seed will produce weak results.

The experience of creating your future and achieving your goals is a lot like that of the farmer and their crop. There is a checklist of items you must be aware of to make sure you are completely harnessing the power available to you. The seed in this metaphor is your intention, and like the seed the farmer plants in the hope of growing a healthy, bountiful crop, your intention must be strong.

There are no shortcuts to this process. This does not mean you cannot shorten or "collapse" time and make your dreams or goals a reality faster than in the past. What it means is that if any of the necessary understandings are not in place, the experiences you want will have a low probability of manifesting. If, by chance, what you want does manifest and any of these important understandings are not met, the experience will not last long. Many people have the ability to create their desired reality at will but don't know how to keep what they create. They fall victim to hidden (or subconscious) mental limitations that eventually surface and seek to destroy any new success that doesn't fit within confines of these limits.

> "Pray that success will not come any faster
> than you're able to endure it."
> —Elbert Hubbard

Achieving an invincible mindset requires a clear understanding of how you influence the creation of your life experiences. When you develop this degree of self-awareness, your actions will demonstrate this clarity as you become wide open to learning what it takes to make your dream come to fruition. Each new action you take involves a new learning process. Each lesson helps you get closer to living the reality you imagined.

The ultimate goal of the invincible mindset is not to *think* you will manifest what you want. It is to *know* you will manifest it. This knowledge cannot be faked. It must be a knowing beyond all thinking. It must be a true state of being: "I AM."

THE KEY TO DISCOVERING YOUR BELIEFS IS SELF-REFLECTION

Since so many of the beliefs or truths that form your identity are subconscious, one of the fundamental keys to next-level mindfulness is self-reflecting and turning what has been a subconscious code that has been running your mind (and limiting you) into a conscious one that serves your intentions. So many people walk around unconscious of the hows and whys of their life. They have never been taught how vital their beliefs and perceptions are to every aspect of their experience. Truly "waking up" is about taking conscious control of the formerly subconscious process that determines how circumstances come together.

Taking any new action that seeks to expand who you are can immediately reveal any hidden mental limits. When thinking about a promotion at work, you might be limited by the idea that you're not good enough to talk to your boss and advance your career any further. When thinking about asking someone out on a date, you might be limited by fears that cause you to be unwilling to take an action that makes you feel vulnerable to rejection. When looking to improve your financial situation, you might be limited by ideas about why you don't deserve a new level of abundance, and you therefore might not act on the opportunities presented to you. You will eventually find the red line of your comfort zone and the limits of what you see as possible as new thoughts and actions challenge old beliefs.

It doesn't matter what you think, what you want, or what you've done. Your current results and your resulting state of mind will reveal what you really have believed.

ALIGNING YOUR TRUTH WITH YOUR DESIRED REALITY

Each step you take toward what you desire will demonstrate what you believe is true. The creative power (or will) behind each step is based on the strength of your personal beliefs. This is why relatively few people have been able to ascend to the success they really want. This is why so many across the world live in a predominant state of mental suffering. They end up stymied by the limitations they hold in their conscious or subconscious minds.

No matter what you want or how hard you work for it, your truth has to be aligned with what you desire in order for your intention to carry the power to create it. Your truth also has to be aligned with what you desire in order to emit the correct frequency of energy to which the universe will respond with the conditions to help make your dreams come true. If the truth you are telegraphing is not producing the right frequency, instead of responding with the right conditions, the universe will respond with the right lesson of awareness.

You cannot fool the universe.

You can't create a passionate, deep, loving, and lasting relationship without having learned to love yourself, believe you can be loved, and feel safe being truly vulnerable with others.

You can't achieve peak performance and the talent to be a

consistent champion when deep down you doubt your ability or believe you're not as deserving as the other competitors.

You can't create financial abundance when you don't believe it's possible for someone like you to be wealthy or you don't see yourself worthy of the responsibility and the joy of money.

You can't create peace in your soul when your truth tells you your fears are real, you let pessimism dominate your thinking, or you keep surrounding yourself with negative people.

THE COMPONENTS OF CONSCIOUS CHANGE

There are five key components in the process of creating what you want. How successfully and quickly you will be able to accomplish your goals is based on how seamlessly you move through this process. Any hesitation immediately reveals a limit in your mind that is holding you back.

When I work with anyone who desires a breakthrough, I ask them specific questions about each of these components to help them reflect and discover what may be impeding their success. These same questions will help you reveal any sticking points and where you might find any limits on what you believe is possible.

Take some time to reflect on each of these questions as it relates to your life. I suggest writing your answers in a journal or on a sheet of paper.

1. **Dream/Desire: Have you clearly defined what you want?**

   The dream you dream will only be big enough and will only be clear to you if you can see it in your mind as attainable. Envision it as clearly as you can and with as much detail as possible.

2. **Intention/Will: Have you focused on taking any willful action toward what you desire?**

   You will only harness your focus and intention and begin to move forward if you think this is possible for you. Otherwise, besides dreaming of your goals, there will be no serious thoughts of "How?" that lead you toward creating or manifesting the dream. Without a strong will, there is no demonstration of the necessary drive and energy to fuel your actions.

3. **Belief: Do your belief structure and personal truth support your actions?** This is truly where the rubber meets the road. You will only infuse the authentic energy of creation into your actions if you have a true passion for what you want and have little or no doubt that what you are doing can be achieved. It's not just your actions that have creative power. Action without belief is based on spiritually empty energy. Action infused with a mindset that has no doubt in the desired outcome allows you to fully commit and gives your energy its true creative power.

4. **Reflection: Are you willing to risk failing, and are you humble enough to always reflect upon what you need to learn?**

   You will only be open to reflection, truth, and learning if your passion to learn and achieve your intent *outweighs your fear of being wrong.* This includes fear of failing or being embarrassed. Humility opens the flow of knowledge that you will need to be successful.

5. **Reaction: Is your identity sufficiently aligned with your goal to keep you persistent in achieving your goal?**

   You will only be relentless and persevere through every challenge and obstacle if your "I AM ..." statements are aligned with what it takes to create what you want. Knowing you will achieve the outcome you desire must be an unshakable truth. Life will challenge you. Challenges will be a great opportunity to demonstrate who you are.

Keep in mind, if you answered no to any of these questions, there is a limit to what you believe is possible for yourself.

Because creation is exact, each step on your path to achieve success must be vetted by life for its authenticity. No one escapes this process. Life is tuning to the frequency of your energy. Your beliefs generate an energetic frequency that is emitted with a certain strength and amplitude. The stronger the belief, the higher the frequency and vibration. The higher the frequency and vibration, the more fluid, timeless, and seamless each step in the process of creation is. The weaker the energy of belief, the lower the frequency and vibration, and the more negative, heavy, and limiting your thoughts are. A lower frequency equates to a more limited or conflict-ridden experience of life. The manifestation of your desires does not occur. The result is *time*!

The way you look at yourself and life produces a certain quality of energy. Like a radio tower, you beam a frequency, signal, wavelength, and overall character of energy out to everyone in your reality. The broad message this invisible energy is radiating is "This is who I AM, and this is what I'm looking to experience." Life simply looks to match this energy with what will be best suited to validate who you are and what you believe is true. You must be careful what you believe or what you're looking for in the world, because you're likely to find it.

Just think about the people in your life who are generally negative, are always causing drama, or have an endless string of troubling things happening to them. It seems like chaos follows them and they can't get out of their own way.

On the other hand, there are people in your life who have a calm, generally positive disposition and seem to glide through life easily, without any strife. At the core of your behavior and what you attract in your life are the deep truths you hold about yourself. This is how critical it is to be aware and in control of your thoughts and beliefs. This is how important it is to be conscious of the quality of the energy you're putting out to your world. This is what it means to be on the path of next-level mindfulness.

HOW SELF-ESTIMATION RELATES TO PERSONAL POSSIBILITY

How do you truly view yourself? Think of a number on a scale of one to ten that represents a combination of how you feel about yourself and how satisfied you are with your current situation in life right now. On this scale, one represents self-hatred and disgust, and ten represents absolute love and perfection. What number on this scale would you assign to yourself in this moment?

Write that number down now. _____

The number you wrote down indicates how available you are making yourself to the field of infinite possibilities. Using the analogy of the size of a bubble or a sphere to represent a measure of these possibilities, here's how they would visually scale.

If you feel like a **one or two** on the scale, your "bubble of possibilities" is about the size of a golf ball or baseball. A bubble this small indicates the belief in an extremely small vision of what is possible. A person with this kind of identity often feels a sense of worthlessness and views themselves (and their life) in an extremely negative way. Homelessness, the inability to care for themselves, trauma, disease, and abuse may be a part of life for a person who ranks themselves and their life as a one or two. Those who are deeply self-deprecating and feel a sense of self-loathing experience a lot of stress. This mindset put them into a near-constant fight-or-flight state. Their energy is mainly used on the fight for daily survival.

If you feel like a **three or four** on this scale, your bubble of possibilities would be more expansive, about the size of a basketball or beach ball. There are a few good things in your life and you have a few glimpses of joy, but it is mainly a life filled with drama and struggle. Negativity and pessimism rule your mind. Life is generally dominated by fear and worry, with little hope or optimism. Conflict is seen as normal, and you are drawn to negative people, negative media programing, and negative experiences. You may achieve your goals, but you don't experience any lasting fulfillment from them.

If you feel like a **five or six** on the scale, your bubble of possibilities is more like the size of a hot-air balloon or blimp. Part of your life is good, joy filled, and fulfilling, but just when things get too good for too long, a negative experience creeps back in and pulls you to the other side of the ledger. You can envision big dreams, but the path to them is still more of a struggle than you'd like. You are on the fulcrum, always swinging from one side of what is possible to the other. Things go from happy and peaceful one minute to sad and pessimistic the next.

If you feel like a **seven or even an eight** on the scale, the expanse of your vision, belief, and actions is much bigger. The bubble of possibilities you live in has expanded exponentially to the size of the moon or the earth on this scale. You view yourself in a mostly loving and positive way. Your experience of life is fun a majority of the time and you're generally in really good spirits. You create much of what you envision for yourself in terms of relationships and business, and you are fulfilled by these experiences. The occasional drama occurs, but negative experiences are rare, and positive experiences, including feelings of optimism and success, are more frequent. There's very little you do not see as available and possible if you put your mind and actions toward it. You consistently magnetize helpful people and positive energy into your life.

If you feel like a **nine**, your bubble of possibilities would be as big the sun. Almost nothing seems impossible. You see yourself with unrestricted, unconditional love and have a sense of unlimited worth. You take action toward your dreams without hesitation, and the world clears a path for you. The right people, places, and information flow to you. Life is joyous, peaceful, and fulfilling. While there are moments of grief and struggle, they are few and far between as life favors you abundantly.

I have never had anyone honestly tell me they feel like a **ten** when reflecting on who they are. A ten has no bubble. There are no limits. There is only pure love and infinite, timeless creation.

This visual scale is presented to clarify the point that you can usually only see, believe, and draw toward yourself what you feel worthy of experiencing. *How you look at who you are is critical because it relates to what possibilities you make available to yourself.* Seeing yourself differently massively expands the opportunities life will bring your way. There is an extremely low probability that someone who views themselves as a three on the scale can experience the same results as someone who views themselves as an eight. The magnitudes of the self-created possibility fields are dramatically different.

In cases where individuals create very successful experiences but on some deep internal level don't feel worthy of this success, they eventually work to destroy it. Your truth always has the last word on your experience and state of mind. There are endless examples in pop culture of very successful actors, musicians, and athletes who achieved high levels of fame, success, and wealth but ended up sabotaging their success by making puzzling and destructive choices. What really happened is that a portion of their identity simply couldn't support the magnitude of what they created. Their ego had no choice but to serve a limiting belief and wreck their opportunities or a good portion of what they created.

LIBERATING YOUR MIND FROM LIMITS

There is a fine line between living the life of your dreams and staying in suffering and want. That fine line lies in how you look at who you are. Change the way you see yourself from incapable to capable, and watch what starts to happen each day. Change your mindset from regretful and shameful to appreciative and feeling good about who you are in this moment, and see how life begins to respond. These are subtle but powerful internal shifts in personal truth. When these shifts are authentic, they can change everything for you. For these shifts to be authentic, you must discover and dismantle all your conscious and subconscious limiting beliefs.

Consider this fundamental and potentially life-changing truth:

Any thought that causes suffering or reflects on you in any limiting or self-denigrating way is a lie or stems from a lie.

There is no limitation on who you really are. This concept may contradict what you have thought or believed for years. It doesn't make it any less true. What is true is your unlimited nature in this moment. Limiting or denigrating thoughts are a lie because they assume you are who you were or that change can't happen. The invincible mind grounds itself in the truth of infinite possibility and in a capable and worthy soul. It doesn't matter if that possibility has a fraction of a percent chance of happening. If it is a positive possibility that will help you achieve what you desire, stay *open* to it. This is a path that allows your dreams to become your reality!

Since self-acceptance, respect, and self-love move you closer to what you want in life, the trillion-dollar question is: "What prevents this beautiful empowering energy from flowing into your mind every day?" As revealed in step two of this book, the nurturing, personal experiences and genetics that have shaped your identity may have left you with many limiting thoughts you simply may have never questioned before. You accepted them as the truth because you didn't know any different. They were subconsciously embedded in your belief system, creating boundaries about who you are and what you can and cannot do. Not anymore.

REMOVING TOXIC AND DESTRUCTIVE LIES FROM THE MIND

To clear the way for you to see and feel more of the *truth of who you really are*, let's examine three of the most damaging concepts of mind that severely limit your creative power. Three of the most self-limiting concepts and emotions are regret, guilt, and shame.

These counterproductive beliefs and emotions create barriers, preventing your mind and spirit from advancing to a fuller expression of who you are. They have limited your bubble of possibilities, and if you carry them into your present and future, they will continually work to restrict you from a more joyful experience of life.

The Lie of Regret

Lingering regret is a concept that represents a denial of the truth and keeps you stuck in personal disdain while hindering your confidence and ability to move forward. Holding regret in your mind from a previous action, past the point of immediate reflection and learning, can do damage to your identity in a number of ways. First, it can make you feel fearful or incapable of trying again without assuming you'll make another mistake and feel additional regret. This is not true. Anything is possible in the next moment.

Second, regret lies to you by causing you to dwell on thoughts about what you "woulda, coulda, or shoulda" done differently. There is only what you did. Accept it and learn from it. If you could have or should have acted differently or better in some past moment, *you would have.* At that moment in time, you did the best you could. That is the self-evident truth. If your mind is fighting you on this truth, watch closely. If your ego is using "would have, could have, or should have," *it is lying to you to hold you back from more of what is possible.* Regret poisons and devalues your identity by causing you to believe "I AM regretful." With this declaration coding your identity, your ego will have no choice but to create more acts of regret.

If you want to embrace more of your creative power, stop focusing on what you regret and start focusing on who you choose to be now! What did you learn that can help you moving forward? Feeling regret for a brief moment is important because it helps you understand who you don't want to be anymore. You cannot go back and change the past. Free yourself now by making the commitment to make peace with every one of your previous actions. This is how you move to the highest state of mind.

The Lie of Guilt

Holding on to feelings of guilt about anything in your past causes negativity, self-loathing, and feelings of unworthiness. The result is a false personal belief that corrodes your identity and limits your future.

Feelings of guilt are important only for the initial awareness they give you of the thoughts and actions you *no longer want to embrace as part of who you are*. However, there is absolutely zero value in holding on to feelings of guilt past this initial response and reflection. Although the world may tell you that you "should" feel guilty, beyond the importance of understanding what you did, carrying guilt into your future is highly corrosive to your self-worth. While you may have thought that feeling bad promotes a positive change in your behavior, it actually does the opposite. It poisons your mindset and devalues your self-image, creating the belief and identity "I AM guilty." With this coding, your ego has no choice but to direct your thoughts and actions in a way that will make you feel guilty again.

I want to be very clear here in distinguishing between the statement "I AM guilty," when it means taking responsibility and acknowledging a past action, and the statement "I AM guilty," when it means feeling unworthy because of a belief you've adopted as a result of that action. Take responsibility for your previous undesired actions, but choose to no longer poison your mind and soul with thoughts of unworthiness due to feelings of guilt. The act that created the guilt came from *who you were*. You have the ability in this moment to define *who you are*. You can renew the spirit of your mind and soul, give yourself grace and forgiveness, and declare a new you in this moment. In this moment you have absolutely nothing to feel guilty about.

The Lie of Shame

Experiencing shame by feeling unworthy, humiliated, and valueless, either because of your own actions or because you allowed someone else to make you feel shameful, is the most effective way to constrict your soul and limit your sense of fulfillment and joy. Carrying shame throughout your life causes incalculable damage to your state of mind and limits your potential.

Of the three most self-limiting concepts (regret, guilt, and shame), shame is the most damaging to your identity. Shame is like regret and guilt to the extreme. Other than as an initial feeling to foster reflection on what caused the reaction of shame and what thoughts, behaviors, or actions you want to avoid in the future, shame has no value. For example, if you harmed someone with your words or actions, the shame would serve you by encouraging you to avoid behaving like that again. Or if you felt shame because someone had become more successful than you, the shame would serve you by reminding you to never let the act of comparison affect how you feel about who you are, no matter how your parents shamed you into believing you need to be successful to be valued. Carrying a feeling of shame in your mind severely reduces your sense of self-love and self-respect. It infects the mind with the identity "I AM shameful." With this coding of your identity, your ego will have no choice but to make you feel shameful again.

Living the lie of shame, past the initial moment of reflection, can keep you stuck in pain and misery for years. To liberate yourself is to see that in this moment you can step out of your shame and into a new version of who you are. It comes down to a simple decision of whether or not carrying shame serves you in terms of who you want to be and what you want to experience now. *In this moment, you are a beautiful, perfect human being with unlimited potential in front of you.* In this moment, you have nothing to feel shameful about.

Is it this simple? Yes, it is. There is no rule book on how long you have to punish yourself by feeling regretful, guilty, or shameful. To achieve real change in your life and a mindset of infinite potential, you must liberate yourself to a new sense of worth where you see that so much more is possible. To see that possibility, you must feel worthy of it. To see your worth, you must see that these poisonous concepts do not serve you in any way.

To move to the highest state of mind, you must see that any shame you've carried was based on your past level of awareness. You must embrace this opportunity now to create the shame-free version of yourself that best serves you going forward. You are worth so much more!

REFRAMING PAST CHOICES

The two most important questions you can ask yourself when it comes to any negative or limiting belief are:

- Does this limiting belief serve me and my current intentions?
- Is this negative thought even true?

As you reflect and dig deeper, you will eventually find the answer to both is an unequivocal and emphatic *no*.

A profound way to shift how you look at yourself is through the lens of learning versus not feeling good enough. In sessions with clients, I ask them if they feel bad about themselves because of mistakes they've made. Almost every single person I've asked this question to says yes. Many immediately say, "Of course! I've made too many mistakes to count!" Here's an example of these conversations:

ME: Do you feel like you've made any mistakes in your life?

CLIENT: Yes, I should have been a less harsh and a more supportive parent to my son.

ME: So, why weren't you?

CLIENT: He was very irresponsible and ungrateful, and I had already given him so much money.

ME: Then, how could you have been more loving than you were?

CLIENT: I could have been patient and given him more money.

ME: Then, why didn't you?

CLIENT: Honestly, I didn't have any more money to give him, and I was already so upset at the trouble and mental anguish he'd already caused me and his father.

ME: Then, how could you have possibly given him any more than you did?

CLIENT: Wow. I guess I couldn't have.

ME: You did the best you could have at the time, given the circumstances and the stress you were under. You did more than so many parents could ever hope to do.

CLIENT: I know. You just always want to go back.

ME: The only time you have is now. Operating from a freer mind will help benefit everyone in your family in the most important time you have—now.

CLIENT: You're right . . .

ME: Mistake or learning experience?

CLIENT: It was definitely a learning experience.

Here's another example:

ME: Do you feel like you've made any mistakes in your life?

CLIENT: Yes, my life is full of mistakes.

ME: Give me an example.

CLIENT: I should have stayed in school and finished my degree.

ME: Then, why didn't you?

CLIENT: I thought I was ready to turn pro and enter the real world and make money.

ME: Then, how could you have stayed?

CLIENT: I could have made a different choice.

ME: Then, why didn't you?

CLIENT: I was broke and tired of the bad energy and coaching politics and was just ready to move on.

ME: Then, how could you have stayed?

CLIENT: I could have put up with it for one more year.

ME: Then, why didn't you?

CLIENT: I don't know, I just felt like I needed to move on.

ME: Then, how could you have stayed?

CLIENT: [Silence] I don't know, I guess I couldn't have at that time.

ME: Exactly. Mistake or learning experience?

CLIENT: I guess when you say it like that, it was a learning experience.

Here is one more example to consider:

ME: Have you made any mistakes in your life?

CLIENT: Yeah, hasn't everybody?

ME: Give me an example.

CLIENT: OK, here's a big one. I shouldn't have cheated during my marriage.

ME: Then, why didn't you not cheat?

CLIENT: I don't know, I was feeling desperate for attention, connection, passion. It just happened.

ME: Then, how could you have not cheated?

CLIENT: Ummm, I could have had some fucking discipline. Ya know, stuck to my vows.

ME: Then, why didn't you have discipline and stick to your vows?

CLIENT: Because I was weak of mind, and starved of intimacy.

ME: Then, how could you have had discipline and stuck to your vows?

CLIENT: What? I don't know, I could have been a better person!

ME: Then, why weren't you, as you say, "a better person"?

CLIENT: I told you. Because I was feeling unwanted!

ME: Then, how could you have not cheated?

CLIENT: I could have . . . I . . . I don't know. [Silence] I couldn't have?

ME: Nope. Not at that time in your life, anyway.

CLIENT: So you're saying it's OK that I cheated?

ME: No, not at all. I am not condoning affairs while in a

marriage or in any committed relationship. I'm simply pointing out the undeniable truth that those decisions reflected the best of your ability at that time in your life. To carry guilt or regret about it serves you in no way. Do you still feel guilt and regret today?

CLIENT: Yes, every day. It sucks.

ME: And remind me again how that negative energy of guilt and regret helps you with what you want to achieve in your life now?

CLIENT: I don't know, it certainly doesn't feel like it helps.

ME: It doesn't. That guilt does not serve you; it only limits you. That moment is over. In order to liberate yourself to experience what you want to create now, you must finally forgive yourself. You must see that it was who you were, not who you are or who you can choose to be. You have to see that it was a learning experience based on the best you had emotionally and mentally at the time.

CLIENT: Yeah, but it wasn't right.

ME: Right or wrong is not the issue now. It's about what will help you going forward! Look, you don't have to like what you did and you certainly don't have to condone it. But are you the same person today? Would you choose to do the same thing again when in a committed relationship?

CLIENT: No, never.

ME: Then, isn't it more mentally and spiritually beneficial to see it as a learning experience rather than a mistake that has to haunt you for the rest of your life? What benefit is there in that?

CLIENT: You're right, it was a massive learning experience.

ME: Did you lose something because of that affair?

CLIENT: Yes, my marriage, my self-respect, too many nights of sleep to count . . .

ME: You came here because you wanted to learn how to stop feeling depressed and find love again? Yes?

CLIENT: Yes.

ME: OK, then finally forgive your younger self, and with that forgiveness, make the commitment to be a different person now. Take full responsibility, learn, and move forward. But move forward with more self-understanding and compassion. With more knowledge of how to respect and hold sacred a commitment to another. Take with you a new awareness of how to nurture a loving connection with any future partner every day. This will serve you so much better in creating the life you want and keeping it! But it starts with a renewed sense of self-respect from this moment forward.

For every mistake you think you've ever made, you can use this process of awareness to see a more empowering way of looking at the past. The optimal and liberating view is through the lens of a "learning experience" where you realize you did the best you could have *at that time*.

Framing it this way does not mean you condone any of the actions you took that you don't like. It does not mean you desire those actions to be something you ever experience again.

It does not mean there were not consequences or effects of those actions that you may have already dealt with or will have to deal with at some point in the future. It does not mean your actions were optimal and cannot be improved upon today.

What you are simply and profoundly realizing is that who you were, and what you did in any moment of your past, was based on a previous version of yourself who didn't know any better. Or, if you knew better, the unavoidable truth is that that version of yourself was incapable at the time of doing better. That was simply the inescapable reality of who you were.

Perceived mistakes can gather in the mind and add energy to the poisonous emotions of guilt, shame, and regret over a lifetime. "Learning experiences," on the other hand, while taking away none of the awareness or understanding of your actions, are a more nurturing and kinder way of looking at who you are. This approach is critical to the process of forgiving yourself, liberating your mind and spirit, and, in turn, massively increasing your ability to create positivity in your life.

Looking at your past actions in this way, have you really made any mistakes at all in your life? No, you have not. You, just like every other human being, have gone through an endless array of learning experiences as you have evolved and shed the skin of many past identities and versions of yourself.

Are you the same person you were ten years ago? Five years ago? How about one year ago? No, not even close.

Life is a learning process. What are we all learning? We are learning how to create and survive as desired. We are learning to construct life in a way that sustains our ability to infinitely create rather than working out of misunderstandings that limit or destroy this magical ability.

> **If you want to go through life in a state of grace and you want to know how to embrace an invincible mindset, you must be kinder and more accepting of yourself.**

ACCEPTING YOUR PERFECTION

What do you call something without a single mistake in it? A piece of flawless art, music, or film? A test without a wrong answer?

You call it perfect.

What does that say about you? You have not made a mistake in your entire life. You are as perfect today as when you were born. It doesn't matter what anybody has said to you, what anybody has done to you, or how anyone has made you feel. It doesn't matter what you've done, how you've felt about it, or how you've looked at yourself. The absolute truth is that in this moment, as in every other moment, you are absolutely perfect.

Does perfect mean better than anyone else? No. Does perfect mean optimal in terms of growing and achieving tomorrow? No. Does perfect mean there are no more learning experiences ahead or continuing consequences from past actions? No. What it does mean is that for your entire life, you have been doing the best you could with what you had *at that moment* in terms of thoughts, emotions, and reactions.

The idea of personal perfection can immediately cause people to recoil or scoff. Years of being taught about being wrong, imperfect, sinful, or flawed, along with possibly generations of conditioning around the idea of unworthiness, can cause this idea to feel uncomfortable. It doesn't make the fact that you are perfect any less true.

> **The further you go down the path of life, the more unavoidable the realization of your perfection will become.**

Many of the most renowned teachers throughout history have consistently offered the truth that we are each perfect and complete as we are. It is the realization of this truth that sets the spirit free. Ascension of mind is about understanding how suffering ends when you see more of who you have the potential to become. True glorification comes from the ability to love yourself and see and act on more of the beauty and possibility of who you truly are. This realization has the potential to bring you to head-covering humility.

So much wisdom about life gets lost in translation over years of misinterpretation. Let's take one simple example from a religious text. It's from a well-known and often taught parable in the New Testament, John 8:2–11. The story is of a woman accused of adultery who was about to be stoned. A group of men picked up rocks and were ready to stone the woman they had condemned. Jesus was asked what he thought, and he responded, "He who is without sin among you, let him throw a stone at her first." Immediately, each man put his stone down and walked away. Soon, they were all gone. Jesus turned to the woman and asked, "Woman, where are those accusers of yours? Has no one condemned you?" She said, "No one, sir." "Neither do I condemn you," Jesus said. "Now go and sin no more."

While for centuries the major takeaway has been about not judging others lest you be judged, there is something deeper offered within this parable. By invalidating every accuser's judgment of the woman, Jesus was basically saying, "Other people have no right to judge you, and neither do I." Therefore, you have no one who is holding you in judgment. *You have no one who is telling you who you are.* You are free to decide who you want to be. Free from being labeled by those who, because of their own hypocritical nature, have absolutely no power or authority to label you.

When Jesus liberated the woman from her accusers and judges and those she thought held power over her, she got her power of self-definition back. Maybe for the first time in her life. Through a new way of looking at herself without the judgment of others and, *even more importantly, without self-judgment*, she was "healed" and free to "sin no more." *Sin*, in this case, means making choices out of a misunderstanding or a limited version of who you truly are. This was the healing power behind Christ's words. This is the true liberating wisdom in the parable.

So many false accusers may have had a hand in labeling you throughout your life. So much of your own judgment, negative self-talk, and false narrative could have weighed you down and stifled your experience for years.

However, this is a new moment of opportunity. It's time to shatter the old, debilitating narrative; the harsh, demeaning voice; and the accusers and judges from your past. It's time to drop the negative story that no longer serves you or your dreams. It's time to step into more of the truth of who you really are.

You are not a sinner. You may have held many negative ideas about who you were, causing a past of destructive thoughts, choices, and actions, or what has been considered "sin." However, these past misconceptions do not have to be part of who you are now. You can choose differently. Ironically, dropping any idea that you are a "sinner" in this moment is one of the most important steps you can take to experience your own salvation and liberation of mind.

You are not flawed. You are a perfect creation and a beautiful work of art who, like every other human being, is continually learning and evolving every day. You are exactly where you are supposed to be on your journey right now. Every perceived imperfection is actually a part of your particular process of becoming more authentically you.

You are not unworthy. If you were born into life, you matter. It is that simple and profound. In this moment you are as worthy and as loved by life as any other person in existence. Your existence as matter is the self-evident truth that you matter.

It's time for some real change. It's time to shed the old negativity and doubt and step into a new identity. This is an important moment and an incredible opportunity for you to not only make peace with yourself but also see the new, vast, unlimited horizon of who you can be and what you can accomplish.

> **Nothing is impossible for one who holds no limits in their mind.**

The infinite divine universe is only waiting for you to experience more self-love and harmonize with the truth of unlimited possibility. When there is an alignment of mind with this understanding, you are in the flow of pure creation. You have liberated your mind and, hence, your soul. And in the words of William Shakespeare, "The world becomes your oyster."

STEP 4 REFLECTION QUESTIONS

Answer the following reflection questions to determine if you're ready to move on to step five. If you can't confidently answer every question with yes, write down why you currently feel this way. Keep your responses with those from all preceding steps.

1. Do you understand that all self-deprecating thoughts of imperfection stem from a lie?

2. Do you realize how limits on how you feel about yourself affect the possibilities of what you can experience and maintain for yourself?

3. Do you see why the concepts of guilt, shame, and regret are poisons to your mind?

4. Do you realize that you have not made a mistake in your entire life?

5. Can you see and believe in your moment-by-moment perfection and worth?

Unshackled

Weight I never knew I carried
Chains I thought were real
No longer a silent burden
I can't even explain how I feel

A lifetime of misunderstandings
A dark path where I always seemed to lose
I finally see my true nature
I finally realize I get to choose

There's no more constraint on my expression
I hold the power of my every thought
A life-altering revelation
A web of lies in which I am no longer caught

Unlimited is my new horizon
A million paths I can now take
Whichever one I may decide on
No longer time will I make

I know the potential that is in me
A radiant love that's bursting to come out
Empowered to hold back nothing
My soul finally freed from all doubt.

PART TWO

BREAKTHROUGH

LIBERATING YOUR SOUL TO NEW POSSIBILITIES

How Self-Awareness Empowers You

Emancipate yourselves from mental slavery,
none but ourselves can free our minds.

—Bob Marley

Liberating yourself from any negative or limited thinking is a massive step along your path to the mindset of infinite potential. As you shift the quality of your state of mind, your dominant energy changes. This is an inflection point on the arc of your existence. This positive internal shift holds the power to change so much for you and for those whose energy you interact with on a daily basis. It also has significant implications for your world.

EMBRACING THE NEW YOU

By working to stretch your awareness, not only are you nurturing your mind, body, and soul with positive energy, but you are also uplifting and healing others. You become a beacon of light that gives and shines positive energy, rather than unintentionally draining the energy of those around you. Healing your soul by coming to a greater understanding of who you are contributes to the healing of your world.

Knowing who you are is the true doorway to the power of conscious creation.

You have now awakened to how you connect with the nature of personal creation. In the preceding steps, you revealed that *you* are the author of your story and only you determine how it gets written from this moment forward. The canvas is blank, the possibilities endless. The only question that remains is: Who do you choose to be now?

If you do not know the answer to this question, it is perfectly normal. Most people grow up with an idea implanted in them by their parents or society about who they should be. The path of awakening is also one where you give yourself the space and time to see what emerges now that you have graced yourself with the permission to let your true spirit shine. Your new liberated soul will eventually nudge you in what feels like the perfect direction. Remember, there is no obligation. You choose from a world of possibilities when you are ready.

This new inspiration about who you want to be and what you want to do can be as simple as having the courage to go after a new job, find daily peace, take your athletic ability to the next level, or improve your relationships. Or this new realization could lead you to something even bigger.

When realizing the extent of these new possibilities, it is normal to think on a bigger scale about what you can do. With so many crises going on in the world, common questions people ask are, "What can one person do to help?" or, "How can I help solve world hunger and assist those who are suffering?" or, "What can I do to make the world more peaceful?" While there are many tangible things that can be done, such as volunteering, running for political office, or donating money, the greatest intangible thing you can do is exactly what you are doing right now: working to expand your awareness and raise your consciousness. When you raise your awareness of who you are, which includes more self-appreciation, self-respect, and self-love, you are in effect raising up the collective consciousness of the world.

While this may seem hard to believe, it is nonetheless true. The degree of this impact is impossible to calculate. *Simply know that it is.* Your state of mind and how you look at yourself have a global impact. The ripples of energy from your heart have an unseen domino effect. Your ripple matters! You have no idea how many people have been affected by the caliber of your energy before this moment, and you have no idea how many will be affected by the quality of your energy and the state of consciousness you decide to embrace from this moment forward.

It is never a question of *if* you matter in this world. It is always a question of *how* you will use this gift to choose to matter each day.

How you define yourself is your free will. Just know that this incredibly divine universe will mirror back to you the exact quality of your most dominant energy and state of mind. It will reflect this back to you in your experiences and life circumstances and in what you see and experience on a global stage. Walk around paranoid and angry and you'll find situations and information to make you feel more paranoid and even angrier. Walk around with optimism, joy, and love in your heart and you will find a world that reflects the beauty of this energy back. Regardless of who you've been, one of life's greatest gifts is that no matter what kind of energy you have put out to your world, in this moment, you can choose to change it.

Any time you change your perspective or outlook, it will feel different and even uncomfortable at first. Anything new is supposed to feel different. Your ego may even try to convince you to turn back to your old attitude, where it felt comfortable and safe. Your ego will use every trick in the book to convince you that your new, positive self is a waste of time.

Do not be dismayed.

This is when you truly have an opportunity to demonstrate

a new level of will regarding a new you. This is when it's critical to see how the choices you make will either perpetuate an old, negative story and unwanted pattern or establish a new way of being. This is when a determined will is required to overcome old behaviors and a stubborn ego.

The ego's stubbornness is rooted in its drive to protect you from change and keep you from entering the unknown. It works to prevent you from abandoning your old way of doing things *even though those old ways have not worked for you*. But years of pain and suffering may give you the fortitude you need. Mental exhaustion may finally lead you to leave your comfortable harbor, sail a new sea, and find a new shore. Anxiety about the future may have drained you for so long that you can no longer listen to the lies of "rinse and repeat." This is because you are now wise to the truth of your perfection. You are now ready to become a master of your reality and the writer of your own script. You now know that the possibilities of what you are worthy of creating are far greater than you ever imagined. You are stepping through the liberating doorway of transformation and expanding your mind, knowing a sea of new possibilities is available to you.

Rather than engaging in the previous pattern of arguing with your significant other, you interrupt the old pattern and say, "I care too much about us to argue any longer. Let's talk this out." While every surging emotion tells you to respond with anger and vitriol, this is when next-level mindfulness matters. This is when you have a massive opportunity to choose differently. It is this type of general example that showcases the opportunity to alter the pattern of your life. To define yourself differently, *not just in mind but in action.*

Instead of blaming others or the coach when you don't play to your potential on the course, field, or court, take a different route and take full responsibility for how you played. The minute you feel any animosity, look at it like an opportunity to go where you haven't felt comfortable. Step back and exhibit self-awareness. Ask yourself what you can do better, and seek to learn from the experience. As I tell all my athletes, "Don't get mad—get curious."

Rather than letting your fears take over your mind and put you into the familiar nightly tailspin about what could happen in the future, recognize your fear-based state of mind, take a breath, and begin to fill your mind with positive ideas of what could happen. The opportunity lies in catching the negative thoughts and countering them with hope rooted in the truth that anything is possible in the next moment. Be determined to stay positive. This is the mindset of ultimate respect for the energy of life, God, or the magnificent universe we live in.

Changing your response and behavior may take some time and a consistent conscious effort in the beginning of your quest. Accepting the new moment-by-moment perfection of who you are can be a new and very unfamiliar experience. After all, you could literally be working against evolutionary dynamics, genetics, unconscious instincts, and comfort zones from thousands of years of family familiarity with mental strife, struggle, and suffering. The impact of war, genocide, slavery, family psychoses, plagues, starvation, or abuse in previous generations could be ingrained in your subconscious and may have had a major influence on the way you've looked at the world. This past residue lurks in almost every human being.

> **Regardless of your social genetic coding, with consistent will, belief, and effort you can change it all.**

The optimistic point is that change can happen instantaneously based on your will to overpower the formerly unconscious thoughts and beliefs that no longer serve you, or this change can take a certain amount of time. *Stay with it.* You can compare this change to making a New Year's resolution to get in shape. When you decide on January 1 that you're going to work out more by going to the gym a few days a week, you immediately have a burst of energy. You sign up for a membership at the gym and go a couple of times in January. Then . . . you know the rest of the story.

At first, a change in the habits of your mind requires trust and massive resolve. It must be a one-way door through which you are determined not to go back to your previous story and way of thinking and being. What can be empowering is what you learned in the preceding steps: that there is so much possibility ahead for you and so much you have to offer your world, your significant other, your family, your career, your sport, your business, or your own mind. This knowledge should inspire you to never go back to the old way of thinking that limits you. Again, limits add time between where you are and what you want. Time creates pressure, and pressure creates suffering.

THE POWER OF INFINITE POSSIBILITY

The following sports example shows what can unfold when you operate from the belief and mindset that anything is possible for you.

In 2014 I was brought in for the season to coach mental strength and the power of mindset for Arizona State's football team and staff. To start, I was assigned to work with the special teams unit. Immediate success in that area led me to work with many other offensive and defensive starters on the team. In the third game of the season, star starting quarterback Taylor Kelly suffered a leg injury and was deemed out for the next few games. Backup quarterback Mike Bercovici had to step up and take over the position. Mike had been waiting a long time for his opportunity and was intent on making his debut a great one. After three years of not starting and of playing a backup role, Mike could have chosen to transfer schools and start for another college team. Instead, he chose to stay loyal to Arizona State and wait his turn as the backup quarterback. In the fourth game of the 2014 season, he finally got his chance. This game was not an easy one by any means. It was a Thursday night, nationally televised home game on ESPN against UCLA, the number eleven team in the country at that time.

With only three days to prepare, Mike stepped up admirably, throwing for almost five hundred yards and three touchdowns. However, two costly interceptions and an Arizona State defense that gave up an eye-popping 62 points led to a tough loss. Mike and I started our mental work the following weekend. As an intense competitor, Mike was determined to bounce back with a victory. The next matchup on the schedule was no easier: a road game against USC, ranked number sixteen in the country at the time, in the Colosseum in L.A. This was twenty-five miles from Mike's hometown, where he grew up playing high school football. To say he was determined to win the game is an understatement.

With a week to go, the main focus of our work was preparing Mike to handle any adversity and maintain a mindset of infinite possibility throughout the game. The other focus was his worthiness and readiness to take on this leading role confidently and with the most determined and positive outlook possible. There is no avoiding the reality of facing adversity in sports. One of the major attributes of the best athletes in the world is their ability to deal with adversity, react appropriately, stay focused, and execute at a high level. This is a major part of the test of an athlete's will. I told Mike that there would likely be moments of adversity in the game and that one of the main things I wanted him to remember is that anything is possible. I wanted him to embrace this critical, limitless idea before every snap of the football. Nothing is impossible to a mind that can open to and act on that infinite possibility. We worked on this in practice, and I reiterated it to him throughout the week as the game drew near.

The football game was a back-and-forth battle. In the fourth quarter with two minutes and forty-three seconds remaining in the game, Arizona State found themselves with the ball and trailing by nine points. Mike stepped up on the next play and threw a beautiful pass down the right sideline for a seventy-three-yard touchdown. Arizona State was now only down 2 points with a score of 34–32, but time was running out and they needed the ball back. The defense did a great job and stopped USC's next drive. Arizona State's offense got the ball back on their own twenty-eight-yard line with twenty-three seconds left in the game and no time-outs. It was what anyone who watches sports would deem a daunting situation.

A quick incompletion on the first offensive play left only seventeen seconds remaining in the game. On the next play Mike remained focused and calmly dropped back to pass. He surveyed the field and then threw a perfect pass across the middle of the field that was completed for twenty-seven yards to the USC forty-six-yard line. Mike had to run to the line of scrimmage and immediately spike the football to stop the clock from running out. Now there were only seven seconds left in the game and they were not in field goal range.

On the next play, which Mike knew would likely be the

last play of the game, he broke the huddle and wound up his two arms like windmills to stretch them for what he knew he was about to do. He then got back in shotgun formation to receive the snap. He dropped back to pass, set his feet, and heaved a beautiful pass over fifty yards in the air to the end zone, where receiver Jaelen Strong jumped up and snatched it out of the night sky in front of four USC defenders. There was no time left on the clock.

Touchdown and victory!

And as the announcer on TV said, "A play that will go down in Arizona State history as one of the greatest ever run by the Sun Devils."

So many years of preparation, desire, work, and patience led to that incredible moment. Mike truly willed that team to victory with his self-belief, focused mind, and relentless competitiveness throughout the game. His faith in the possibilities regardless of the adversity he faced dominated the energy of the team and created that entire fourth quarter comeback, all the way down to the last second of the game and the unforgettable miracle play he manifested.

The entire team actually adopted this powerful mindset of possibility that was offered to them throughout the season, and we went on to achieve an outstanding 10–3 record that year. This included a major season- and school-defining victory over eighth-ranked Notre Dame, a national ranking as high as eleven, and a victory over Duke in the Sun Bowl. This was one of the best seasons in the past twenty-seven years of Arizona State football.

When you have that kind of will, and you work to develop the talent necessary, and then you add a mind that only sees what is possible, you have magic. The great part about this story is that you do not have to be an athlete to stretch your mind and energy to embrace infinite possibilities for your life. This state of mind is available and transferable to you for anything you desire to do or experience in the world.

> **You are a limitless creator with unlimited worth and potential. Anything is possible for you. What makes any dream probable depends on the strength of your beliefs, and how determined you are to learn and persist along the road of creating it.**

Accepting unlimited success for yourself based on seeing your unlimited worth can be immediate or it can be a process. Consider this conversation I had with a client:

ME: How are you doing with all this newfound self-belief, self-appreciation, and love?

CLIENT: Honestly, it feels a bit weird, but I'm getting better with it. The perfection thing throws me now and then.

ME: How so?

CLIENT: Isn't it a little narcissistic to say you're perfect? I mean, nobody's perfect.

ME: Then everyone is.

CLIENT: Huh?

ME: If nobody's perfect, then everyone is perfect in their imperfection.

CLIENT: Wow, I'm gonna have to sit with that one for a bit.

ME: Remember, perfect does not mean optimal, and it certainly doesn't mean better than anyone else. It simply means you're doing the best you can in each moment. So keep being kind to yourself. Honest, but kind. It matters when it comes to what's possible for you.

CLIENT: OK, so it's not a prideful or cocky thing?

ME: No, not at all. It's a self-understanding, respect, and compassion thing. Feeling "less than" is the root of all your frustrations and negativity, and it's the reason you haven't had a breakthrough yet toward what you want. You have to genuinely see yourself as worthy in order to create and attract the experience of it. After all, how can the universe grace you with a possibility you don't feel worthy of?

CLIENT: So life just can't give me what I want because I'm a good person and have been through enough suffering in my life?

ME: It's not about how much you've been through or what good deeds you've done. It's about how much you've learned. It's about how you feel about yourself and the possibilities. Everyone's path is different. Life presents lessons until there is no need for the lesson anymore.

CLIENT: Well, I'm tired of all the lessons.

ME: I understand. That's why it's imperative to reflect and redefine yourself not only in terms of who you believe you are and the limits of what you see as possible, but also in terms of how you decide to act and react every day. You have to demonstrate your true will to experience change.

CLIENT: So I have to get comfortable with being uncomfortable?

ME: Bingo. Yes. You have to get comfortable feeling good, acting from optimism, and knowing you not only can do good and give joy, but can create and also receive joy and the things you desire in your life. Given a bit of faith in demonstrating this new version of yourself, you may shock yourself with the results you produce.

CLIENT: And what if this new attitude doesn't change anything?

ME: Then you'll lose absolutely nothing, and actually, you'll gain the self-respect to know you worked to positively change your energy and outlook. In fact, the mentally strong question and optimal thought is, What if it does change everything? This type of mindset change certainly has been the key for thousands who have walked this path before you.

THE POWER OF SELF-UNDERSTANDING

Throughout the process of liberating your mind and stepping into this new version of yourself, you must embrace several key attributes about who you are. Each of these adds fuel to your power of conscious creation.

Self-understanding is the first attribute of personal liberation and a critical part of developing a mindset of infinite possibilities. Through the reflective process of self-understanding, you see the construction of your entire identity up to this moment. When you make this discovery from a place of true curiosity, it moves you to a nonjudgmental state where the reason for every one of your past behaviors becomes crystal clear. You didn't choose your genetics, your place of birth, your economic conditions, your upbringing, your relatives, your religious leaders, or your teachers at school. You trusted those who were older than you and often gave them more credit than they deserved. You thought that because they were in a position of authority or power, they had knowledge that could help you. Sometimes this is true, but many times, unfortunately, it is not.

You did the best you could have to understand yourself and make the choices that allowed you to survive. *The hand you were dealt was not in your control.* How you played the hand as a child and as a teenager was the best way you knew how. With age and experience comes wisdom, and soon you get smarter at playing your hand. You begin to realize you're always going to receive new cards (like right now) and you get better and better at navigating life. This is the evolving nature of who you are. With self-understanding, before you know it, you're dealing yourself your own cards and winning the game of life.

The power in self-understanding lies in the compassion it brings. It is important not to blame the choices you made in your past or your current circumstances on your conditions at birth or your upbringing. Simply understand that this was your unique path to this moment. For a billion reasons you can't know yet, *it was what it was*. The invincible mind works from the faith that there is a reason for everything. Those reasons will reveal themselves at the right moment.

> **Self-understanding is the path to complete forgiveness of yourself and others.**

Acceptance does not mean you condone things you did in your past that don't conform to your current set of values. Acceptance also does not mean you would be OK doing them again. It simply means you are no longer going to fight the truth of your unique journey to this moment. You are just finally accepting that it's a part of who you were. This is mental and spiritual liberation. This is breaking the anchor in your mind of any resisted part of your past and setting yourself free from the suffering of being stuck in the past.

This does not mean you do not honor your heritage. This does not mean you do not honor your culture. This does not mean you do not honor your mother or father (if for no other reason than the fact that they conceived you). It does not mean you throw all your history away. What it does mean is that you are no longer going to resist whatever path it was, and whatever you had to choose to do and endure, that brought you to this moment and this insight now.

Many people go lifetimes without the blessing of

self-awareness and self-understanding. You are here now. Be proud of yourself. Switch the focus of your thinking from what you haven't done or created yet to what you have done and overcome throughout your entire life just to get here. (If there is one shred of resistance to the full acceptance of your unique path of life, I encourage you to revisit part one of this book.)

Part of self-understanding is also an acceptance of your behavior toward others. It enables you to understand why you did what you did and become keenly aware of how this may have had a negative impact on someone else. There may be consequences and, possibly, lasting effects, particularly on the minds of others, that you will have to acknowledge and deal with. However, the memory of the old you will fade in direct proportion to how consistent and genuine you are with the expression of the new you.

An analogous example involves a dog rescued from a shelter. If the dog was neglected or abused by its prior owner, it will be wary of any new interactions. You may raise your hand to pet the dog and the dog may flinch and cower. Its memory of being hurt prevents it from seeing or believing in the new actions from a human. The dog is simply protecting itself based on past interactions.

The same is true of anyone in your life who has interacted with the "old you." They don't know the "new you" yet. It will take some time for people in your life to adjust, especially if they are used to a radically different version of who you were. Regardless, you must choose to make this change, for yourself first and foremost. Some will acknowledge your shift, and some may not. This cannot be your concern. Your responsibility is to be aware of people's possible reactions so you do not experience disappointment, which can throw you off-balance. Stick to the new identity and behavior that serve you, and keep being who you desire to be now.

The path of Robert Downey Jr. is a great pop culture example of how this works. Known globally for his famous role as Tony Stark or Iron Man, he is one of the most well-known, highest-paid, and popular actors of his generation.

It wasn't always this way.

Robert was born in 1965 in New York, and by the time he was five years old, he was already acting. By six he was smoking weed and drinking alcohol with his father. Drug use was common in his household as his mother had problems with alcohol addiction. His parents ultimately divorced in 1978. He then moved with his father to Santa Monica, California, and continued acting. He dropped out of high school at sixteen to pursue acting full-time.

His acting career soon took off with stints in the cast of *Saturday Night Live* and off Broadway. He was even nominated for an Academy Award in 1992 for his incredible leading role in the movie *Chaplin*. In spite of all this success, his drug and alcohol use continued to get much worse. In 1996 he was pulled over and arrested for possession of cocaine and heroin along with a .357 Magnum handgun. For this he was very fortunate to be given only probation. Regardless, his self-destructive behavior continued, and he went on to violate his probation three consecutive times. In 1999 he was finally sentenced to three years in prison.

Robert ultimately entered rehab in 2001 and soon after was arrested again for being under the influence. This got him fired from his TV job on the hit show *Ally McBeal*. He was now out of work and broke, and was ordered back to rehab, yet again. Finally, in 2003, his wife, Susan, gave him a life-changing ultimatum: "Me or the drugs." He then got self-aware and sober for good.

In 2003 Robert got another chance and started steady film work again, and in 2008 he was cast as Tony Stark in *Iron Man*. Since then, he has not looked back and has become one of the most famous and successful actors in Hollywood. In 2024 he achieved even more and won the Academy Award for Best Supporting Actor for his role in *Oppenheimer*. Robert is also a major philanthropist, having donated millions to several charities, including those that help people recover and transition to a new, more positive way of life.

His incredible story of destruction and redemption is a testament to the power of the will to change who you are. Equally as poignant is the demonstration that as you change, the negative memory of who you were fades as well. In the 1990s he was an actor who couldn't stay off drugs and eventually couldn't even get hired because of his chaotic reputation. Now, an entire new generation knows him only for his success as an incredibly talented and extremely popular actor.

The self-understanding that brings consistent change brings with it a new narrative of who you are. Stay patient and consistent on your new path. The world will ultimately adjust and submit to the truth of the new you.

THE POWER OF SELF-FORGIVENESS

The power of self-awareness brings you to the realization that there is nothing to forgive. In this state of clarity, you see the truth of your perfection and hence the world's perfection.

The definition of *forgive* is "to stop feeling angry or resentful for an offense, flaw, or mistake." When you no longer allow yourself to be offended by others, when you no longer see constant imperfection in yourself, and when you no longer believe in any negative ideas about your self-worth due to mistakes, *there is nothing to left to forgive.* An elevated state of mind indeed!

Holding anger or resentment in your mind and body toward another person or yourself has no positive benefit. In fact, it prevents peace of mind and the clarity needed to make smart decisions. Resistance generates negative energy. Basically, any nonacceptance of *what is*, or any lack of ability to understand *why*, results in mental conflict and ultimately produces negative emotion. However, through the process of self-understanding, you can see why and how any resistance and negative energy was generated. By seeing how any undesired experience became a manifested possibility in your life, you can dissolve the mental conflict. No more conflict, no more imbalance of energy. This calm, balanced state makes it much easier to forgive and to let go of your destructive angst, either toward another person, your world, or yourself.

When you hold your own self in contempt, you limit both what you see as possible and your ability to create. Forgiveness liberates your soul from this self-judgment. This frees your mind to allow in new experiences and results.

When I met Mel Reid, she was known as one of the most talented golfers on the LPGA Tour who was still without a victory on the tour. She was a smart, witty Englishwoman with a magnetic personality, the fitness of an Olympic athlete, a mischievous and beautiful smile, and loads of talent. At almost thirty-three years of age, she was facing a point in her career where she was wondering if a victory on the LPGA Tour would ever come.

The road to this point had not been an easy one. A great player since her youth, Mel grew up playing many local tournaments and became one of Britain's most prominent amateurs. She turned pro in 2007 and was Rookie of the Year. She would ultimately win six times on the Ladies European Tour (LET). However, in 2012 her life took a devastating turn when her mother, Joy, on her way to watch Mel play in an event in Germany, was tragically killed in a head-on car crash.

Understandably, this completely turned Mel's world upside down. She went back and forth between playing golf and dealing with the tremendous amount of grief she felt. She also was carrying a heavy burden of guilt, feeling that the accident was somehow her fault. Mel actually found a way to manage that guilt and, as a testament to her talent, win several times in Europe after her mother's passing, but quietly and internally she was still struggling. A self-described rebellious mode and lots of late nights became a distraction from her grief and pain, and her game was suffering because of this. She just wasn't living up to her true potential and personal expectations, and she knew something had to change.

In 2018 she took several major steps in her life. She made the ultimate leap of faith and moved from England to the United States to pursue her dreams on the LPGA Tour. She also took the big step of coming out as gay and used her example of courage and her platform as an athlete to support LGBTQ individuals who were looking for positive role models.

After a rough stretch of many missed cuts in her first year on the LPGA Tour in 2019, she began to look for other answers in her quest for next-level performance. We connected and started working together in August 2020. Mel's tough, playful, and at times antagonistic exterior was partly a mask for her fear of vulnerability on the inside. She was understandably still dealing with an unresolved and heavy burden from the passing of her mother. She still thought that in some way she was responsible for what happened. Because Mel was willing to dedicate herself to opening up, reflecting, and understanding where the pain and, hence, the limits of her mind were coming from, she came to realize a vital new truth: her mother's destiny had nothing to do with her. In other words, her mother's passing was not her fault in any way.

This reflection required determination and a genuine desire to be free of her destructive thoughts and their impact on her mind, her athletic performance, and her daily life. This process took many weeks of talks, but upon the ultimate realization of this truth, she released the weight of the hidden guilt that had affected her for years. Her mind was finally free. She finally felt more deserving and worthy. She was finally ready to let her true world-class talent shine without restriction. These supportive feelings are critical for any human being looking to expand their potential.

Two weeks later, she had the lead going into the final round at the LPGA Portland Classic. Not having been in a contending position in a while, she played great on Sunday but fell just a couple of strokes short of victory and finished in fifth place. In the past, her mind would have used this result as evidence that she was not good enough or was unworthy of winning. This time, with a fresh new sense of self-worth, Mel went into the following week with a smile and a confidence she hadn't felt in years. I remember her distinctly telling me on Sunday night after her final round in Portland, "I can't wait to get to next week!" Get to next week she did, and in October 2020 at the ShopRite LPGA Classic she positioned herself in the final group with a two-stroke lead on Sunday. On the fifteenth hole she had a very lengthy and testy twenty-foot putt for par that was critical to keep her momentum and her lead. She got over the putt and buried it straight in the hole, telling me later, "Howard, I literally willed that putt into the hole." That is exactly what happens when you are living life or creating your experience from a sense of belief in your worthiness, who you are, and what you are doing. Nothing can keep you from your true ability or from demonstrating it. Mel stood on the eighteenth hole with a two-shot lead and finished with a par, putting out for her first LPGA Tour victory. It was a well-deserved and life-changing moment for her.

By facing her fears and having the courage to reflect on a painful experience, Mel liberated her mind. Her newfound sense of personal value dictated a completely new identity and inspired energy that led to a breakthrough experience at the top level in the world. It doesn't matter how hard you work or how much talent you have. If you continue to question your worth or carry any unproductive and heavy burdens of guilt, shame, or regret, these beliefs will continue to have a negative impact on your results. New results can only emerge when you identify, understand, forgive, and let go of these misunderstandings.

THE POWER OF SELF-LOVE

When you fully forgive yourself for anything in your past and you see life as a journey of learning and growing, you simultaneously remove all the reasons not to fully love and appreciate who you are now. You also see the perfection of why you are where you are right now. You are finally free of negative energy that you may have carried for years in your mind, body, and soul. As a result, the frequency of your energy completely reconstitutes. When you have no more thoughts of imperfection or "woulda, coulda, shoulda," you gain a sense of harmony and peace of mind that opens you up to the most powerful energy in the universe: the energy of self-love.

Self-love is the holy grail of all positive creative energy.

Self-love is the key to the door of infinite possibility. It is the bedrock state of consciousness for the way you will look at yourself and your world for the rest of your existence. When you give this kind of nonjudgmental, unconditional love to yourself, you also give this grace to your world. Because what you see in yourself, you see in the world. This type of self-acceptance feels like a warm blanket within which you can simply go forward in the world and know everything else will take care of itself.

This is not an arrogant self-love through which you are trying to force yourself to feel better. This is a genuine understanding that reveals without a doubt that you're good enough for what you desire or dream of experiencing. It is an understanding that you were never worth any less than anyone else. You matter and are equally worthy.

Remember, no matter how uncomfortable it seems at

first to feel this way, the vital act is to *let the love in*. This is the only path to an invincible mind. Self-love is the anchoring piece of the puzzle, and it fuels your presence, your vision, and the power behind the critical actions that will draw every necessary condition into place.

Many people state what they want to accomplish and then work consistently toward the dream. *Few, however, actually achieve the dream*. Why? Because on the self-improvement part of the path, they go through the motions of reading, reflecting, and trying to feel different about themselves for a moment. Or they work with a coach who motivates them for a short period of time, or they go to a seminar that energizes them for a week or so. The minute they forget their value and true power, the old negative thoughts sneak right back into their minds and dominate their actions or nonaction.

When it comes to building the life they desire, what they may not realize is that intention must be supported by the daily sense of worthiness that can only come from a consistent feeling of self-love. Self-love can only come from an understanding of the perfection of each step of the journey and the infinite possibilities available to them in this moment.

Self-love allows you to be limitless in your dreams, hopes, and desires. This love expands your vision without effort or hesitation. It puts a force field in front of you that renders negative thoughts or any idea of limitation powerless over your self-belief. Self-love must be practiced every day because the influence of negativity and limitation lurk around every corner in the world.

Self-love fuels your belief and energizes your will and the actions that move you closer to what you want.

Self-love allows you to trust the circumstances when you are faced with challenges on your path.

Self-love magnetizes this same type of love back to you from your world.

Self-love gives off an aura of peace and knowing that provides comfort, peace, and healing to others around you.

Self-love is the greatest gift you can give yourself and others.

Self-love is the greatest love of all.

PRACTICING SELF-LOVE

Here's a powerful exercise to get more comfortable with this new feeling and energy. Practice sitting with this love and this understanding at least once every day.

Pick a time when you are by yourself in a quiet space, or put noise-canceling headphones on with no music. Sit comfortably, preferably with your back straight up, and close your eyes. Breathe slowly and measuredly. Let all the mental noise and distracting thoughts quiet or just pass through. See these thoughts dissipate, lose energy, and dissolve in your mind like clouds. Begin repeating in your mind on each inhale, "Love, perfection, limitless." Feel the energy of this thought and let the love pervade every cell of your body. Embrace this energy with your in-breath, and on your exhale feel, say, or softly whisper, "I AM love." Then sit for a few beats with that truth. Let any negative energy or doubt go with every exhale. On the next inhale, repeat and stay with this loving feeling for as long as you can. Then exhale out any disharmonious energy.

First, try this silent self-love meditation for three minutes. Set your phone timer and do that now.

No, I'm serious. Right now.

Practice letting go and feeling this for just three minutes. Prove to yourself you are committed to becoming a master of your mind rather than letting your scared, old ego and mind talk you out of it with a million reasons why now is not the time, or that doing this exercise feels uncomfortable. Don't fall for the excuses, and don't read the next paragraph until you are finished with this three-minute meditation to start. I'll wait.

Tomorrow, practice this meditation for five minutes, the next day do it for ten minutes, and keep going until you can do this love meditation at will and for at least thirty minutes or as long as you desire. But commit to doing this self-empowering practice daily.

The purpose of this exercise is to work your mind like any other muscle in your body. Feeling the truth of your worth, and loving and appreciating who you are, is vital to expanding your consciousness. Expanding your consciousness elevates the frequency of your energy. The new, higher-frequency energy you emanate creates new positive experiences in your life. Done properly, this meditation will make you feel more alert, clear, grounded, and peaceful afterward. Ultimately, you'll feel more empowered. *You deserve these powerful minutes each day.*

If doing a meditation like this is new to you, it is really important that you stick with it and make it part of your routine every day. Meditating on this thought cannot be a one-time deal. Change does not happen that way. Authenticity and consistency are the keys to real change and lasting transformation. It's a matter of will.

THE POWER OF SELF-BELIEF

While understanding, accepting, and loving yourself is the rocket fuel of creation, self-belief is the engine of your actions. With self-belief, you act with an energy that nourishes your dreams and desires. It is a tangible energy that works to magnetize the conditions needed for what you want in your life.

Much of what you've created in your life has required you to have some level of self-belief. However, your belief must be strong enough now to keep you focused and consistent. You have to have the resiliency to push through the inevitable experiences that will test you before you break through to a new level of being and get the job done. You must be strong enough to keep persisting.

You have to keep going on dates until the person who finally feels right for you shows up.

You have to keep working on your athletic talent and competing until the momentum happens or the victory finally occurs.

You have to keep trying new jobs until the vocation that fulfills your soul emerges as your path.

You have to keep asking questions until the answers that bring you true peace finally show up and enter your mind.

When you see and feel your true unlimited worth, your beliefs become strong enough to create miracles in your life.

I grew up in a financially unstable household, and it was clear that many of the problems my parents were dealing with in their relationship involved money. During my childhood, they separated a few times. They ultimately divorced when I was in my midtwenties. Because of what I witnessed growing up, when I decided to go to college, I chose to center my studies on finance. My thought process was that I'd get my arms around the issue of finances so I wouldn't have the same problems my parents did. So, upon graduation from college (which seems like three lifetimes ago), I got a job in the finance industry. I started as an assistant to an investment representative and then became an investment representative myself.

I worked long hours while making very little money in those days. I was working on my business and building a clientele from scratch, which took a lot of time and patience. One day, an idea crossed my mind that came from a scene in *Wall Street*, a movie I'd recently seen. In the scene, Bud Fox, a young stockbroker played by Charlie Sheen, finally lands the big, life-changing client Gordon Gekko, played by Michael Douglas. They meet for lunch, and as Gordon Gekko gets up to leave, he hands Bud Fox a check to open an account for a million dollars. As a young man who'd been trying to make it in the world on my own since I was seventeen, the scene left an impression on me. *Wouldn't that be cool someday?* I thought.

About a year later, I became familiar with a company that I thought was a great growth stock idea. So, after doing some research and visiting the company, I began presenting the idea to clients. One day, I thought, *Why not take this unique, seemingly undiscovered idea and present it to the biggest technology or growth investors in the world?* I believed in the investment idea, and I believed in me. (I was also naive enough to believe I could accomplish this feat.) I went to the library; got my hands on an old, six-inch-thick Moody's reference book of the biggest growth funds in the world; and found the phone numbers for the biggest tech and growth funds in the country. When I got back to the office, I began dialing. My hope was to get a fund manager on the phone to whom I could present the idea and see if I could get an order and open an account with them.

I dialed and dialed and dialed every day for a month straight. When my coworkers found out what I was doing, they literally laughed at me. They told me I was crazy and that no big mutual fund manager in New York was going to listen to some young stockbroker at a small firm in Arizona. They said it was hopeless and I was a fool for trying.

Thankfully, my belief and my optimism held firm. I continued on my quest. Most of the time, when I called a fund, I was stopped by the gatekeeper, who would tell me the manager was too busy to speak with me, but if I wanted to send some information, I could. I followed the protocol, sent a package of information with my card, and put a note on my calendar to follow up in a week or so.

A month into my attempt, I still had no results and started to wonder if I was a little overambitious. Working to accomplish this was a tall order, but I *believed* in the idea and I really *believed* I could do this. I also knew that these particular types of managers were always on the lookout for an undiscovered company with great technology and promise, so I continued to work at it every single day, undeterred by the roadblocks, the rejections, and the terrible ridicule from my coworkers.

Then, one afternoon, in the middle of probably my twentieth follow-up call of the day, the fund manager from one of the biggest technology growth mutual funds in the world picked up the phone. For a moment I froze and was caught off guard by actually getting through to the head guy. He said, "Hey Howard, I took a look at the company you sent the information about and I really like the idea. I'll start with a hundred thousand."

My heart felt like it stopped. Actually, time felt like it stopped.

I replayed what he had just said in my head, gathered myself, and looked at the stock price on my computer screen. The stock was trading at 10¼. I swallowed, took a deep breath, and then slowly asked, "Do you mean dollars or shares?"—knowing full well the major difference his answer would mean.

He replied, "Shares. I'll start with a hundred thousand shares and then add to it from there."

I immediately did the math. A hundred thousand shares times 10¼ is $1,025,000. I shut my eyes and smiled for just a second as I breathed in and let the reality of what just happened sink in. My mind wandered off. A million-dollar order . . . I did it . . . Quickly, I snapped back to the call and said, "Yes sir, I'll start the order right now and call you when it's completed."

I was in my midtwenties at the time. This was a really big deal for a number of reasons, the least of which were financial. What I was most proud of was setting my mind to accomplishing this big goal and not listening to the negativity and naysayers around me. I stayed focused on what I believed was possible. At that time in my life, my optimism and my belief about what I could do got a priceless boost, which paid many "belief" dividends for years to come. Was my patience tested? Yes, absolutely. Could all that work have been for nothing? Yes. But I stayed present in my belief of what could happen and did not waver as I went through the process. I learned what I needed to know to navigate toward the goal and give it the best chance of happening, and I kept going. This experience gave me the confidence that contributed to many significant personal accomplishments in the days and years ahead.

When striving for your dreams and desires, you have to stay focused on what you believe is possible. You cannot listen to anyone else who comes from a different perspective and a place of limited thinking. And here's an unfortunate truth: most people do come from this limited place. You must stay focused on what *you know* can happen. You must stay in the process. You must stay open to learning what you need to know to increase the probability of success. You must have a will that never gives up. If I gave up years ago, the wonderful experience that led to the insights in this book would have never happened.

> **Belief in yourself, combined with clear intention and relentless perseverance, is the most powerful recipe for manifesting what you desire to experience.**

Self-belief is a critical part of the invincible mindset. It fuels your actions and the tangible energy that is felt by everyone around you. It becomes the magnet for your desires.

It determines how you treat yourself and, in turn, how the world will treat you.

THE POWER OF SELF-RESPECT AND SELF-WORTH

Self-belief produces a feeling of worth, and a feeling of worth produces a mindset of self-respect. Before realizing your true, unlimited worth, you may have had some self-doubt and insecurities that led to a lack of self-worth or a lack of self-respect in certain ways.

Not anymore.

Your new understanding of yourself and the empowerment and mastery of mind that it brings automatically lead you to respect and honor yourself. In more direct terms, this understanding makes you feel like a queen of queens or a king of kings in terms of self-respect and honor. This is a moment of self-realization when you see yourself as a divine creation born of a divine universe. There are no imperfections from a universal perspective—only moment-by-moment creative perfection. This creation includes you.

Why not you?

If you truly see yourself this way, you will keep your mind focused on only the highest thoughts, the highest choices, and the highest actions. The high road will be the only one you ever travel. This is where the conscious state of flow emanates from. This is the mindset and energy of divine grace.

You have stepped into the highest version of the highest vision you have for yourself.

You can now fully harness the creative process of life. Prior to this level of self-understanding, you may have known the creative process but not fueled it with enough self-worth to even spark the engine. It may have consisted of a lot of wanting, envisioning, and working without results. Or you may have created what you want but it didn't last. To consciously create your life in a way that leads to lasting fulfillment, joy, and success, self-worth and love must be unlimited.

Below is a personal declaration that summarizes the self-realization of the first five steps in the journey toward an invincible mindset. These statements of truth are what elevate your mind and soul to align with the success you desire.

Read this declaration and embrace every line as deep in your soul as you can. This is your mantra of personal liberation. This is rocket fuel for your creative process!

PERSONAL DECLARATION

In this moment, I grant myself the permission to be open to and embrace a new idea of who **I AM**.

I take full responsibility for the decisions in my life that have led me to this sacred moment. I choose to do this without any guilt, shame, or regret, understanding that in each past moment, I did the best that I could at that particular moment in time. I understand that everyone is doing the best they can in their own way as well.

While I may not condone some of the actions that I or others took previously, nor would I choose them again, I will draw upon the wisdom gained from these experiences to make new, more empowered choices now.

I AM learning that every experience I have gone through during my life has served me in some way. Therefore, I choose to accept and be grateful for everything and everyone in my life who is allowing me to learn. I understand that in each moment, the elegant universe is always presenting me with exactly what I need to learn and accept in order to move closer to what I truly desire to experience.

I AM worthy of peace, happiness, love, and the creative vision I imagine for myself. I now realize that any idea of personal imperfection, lack, or limitation is an illusion. This is an illusion that I no longer choose to maintain; rather, I choose to set myself free to a life of unlimited possibility.

I AM not who I was ten years ago, one week ago, or even five minutes ago. **I AM** who I decide to be right *now*. This choice is my greatest power.

While I may have many new learning experiences along the way to what I want to achieve, I will eventually succeed because I have become fully aware of how to honor, respect, and love the true creative perfection that **I AM.**

EMBRACING THE POWER OF "I AM"

How to Own the Sacred Narrative of Your Life

Shine like the universe is yours.

—Rumi

If there is a phrase that encapsulates the energy behind every incarnation in the known universe, it is the statement "I AM."

"I AM" is one of the shortest sentences in the written word, but the one that holds the most power—because what you believe, feel, and speak about who you are shapes every moment of your life.

Your "I AM" thoughts and statements are the actual building blocks of how things come together along your journey. They are the nucleus, or the source code, of your identity, because they become the instructions for your ego in terms of what it will work to create, protect, defend, and validate. Your "I AM" statements emanate from beliefs you hold both consciously and, even more powerfully, subconsciously about who you are.

Sometimes, our core beliefs are oppositional and are out of alignment with who we think we are. Here's a simple example. Let's say you think of yourself as a confident person, but deep within you, you hold the "I AM" belief "I AM not good enough." And let's also say that periodically your confidence is shaken, and you know it—you just don't know why. You often hold yourself back from taking steps that would move you forward in different areas of your life. The reason is that this limiting "I AM" belief you've let live in your mind unchallenged has overridden your most well-intentioned plans. If this "I AM" declaration has become your truth, it will have a significant influence on your results *until you change that truth.*

As I explain in step three, the ego's job is to validate what you believe is true about yourself and your world. In essence, this is the feeling of *being* or *existing.* This validation can come from a tangible experience in which the outside world confirms your truth (your "I AM" belief). Alternatively, the mental acceptance can be an internal one where the ego convinces your mind your beliefs are true ("I AM") without outside validation.

The ego takes the path of least resistance to protect and validate your beliefs. Your ego will use whatever belief works to bring you to a state of peace, whether the belief is true or not.

You can believe you're one of the greatest singers in the world. This can work as your truth until you decide to test it by some measure. One way is going to the auditions for the reality TV show *American Idol*. If the director puts you in front of the judges, you will find out very quickly whether or not you are one of the greatest singers in the world outside your own mind and ego.

Keep in mind that all delusion (ignorance of truth) is destined to lead you to another learning experience. It is life's divine way of moving you more in line with universal truth and therefore increasing your probability of survival. Your ego's tricks to avoid truth will only last so long as the reality of what is really true (facts) keeps coming at you. Your ego can be resistant to helpful truth in many circumstances: at your job, in your relationship, on your path to athletic success, when running a business, when trying to find purpose, and when searching for spiritual insight. Millions of people move from delusion to delusion to protect what they want to believe is true in order to avoid fear, guilt, shame, or regret. This only extends the time it takes to achieve your goals and desires *and, ironically, prolongs your suffering*. The key to being open to truth is building up a sense of faith in yourself to the point where you don't fear being wrong or feel bad about being previously unaware. Supreme humility is a powerful way of living, and it is why an invincible mindset has been achieved only by those who are not faint of heart. It is truly a narrow path.

HOW YOUR IDENTITY WORKS WITH YOUR EXPERIENCE

The fastest path to peace and true empowerment is to align your "I AM" statements with the acceptance of truth in every moment.

Living in harmony with the truth is not the challenge. The challenge is that to do so, one must have the willpower and the courage to change what one has believed to be true.

When we make changes in behavior, choices, or attitude that do not come from a true change in identity, they end up being short-term changes. For lasting change, you must be able to consciously break the pattern of habitual negative thinking and become dedicated to a consistently positive way of living. Your willpower and courage must be cultivated into a *relentless pursuit of truth* above all else so you can rise above past negative habits and patterns and demonstrate a new, beautiful understanding of infinite potential and possibility.

You must be unyielding in your determination to be this new version of yourself ("I AM").

Consider the following example of a defining statement, an experience, and the ego's reactions:

Defining statement: "I AM smart with money."

Tangible experience: You lose money on a bad business venture, investment, or career move.

Ego's reactions: If your ego does not want to let go of the belief "I AM smart with money," it will work to protect the belief. Your ego will immediately begin rationalizing why the loss wasn't your fault. Your ego will cause you to lie to yourself until you are convinced you didn't do anything to cause the loss. You may demonize other people, the economy, the market, or anything else to deflect responsibility and keep on feeling you are smart with money.

This example demonstrates how the ego can continue to lie to you to protect a belief that is in peril. The problem with self-protection or denial is that you learn nothing through the experience. You'll be destined to harsh money-losing lessons until your will for change causes your ego to accept that you were not smart with money (past tense). Once you finally accept this truth, you can finally learn how to *be* smart with money and begin to make new choices. By doing so, you can create a belief that is now in line with the truth "I AM learning to be smarter with my money." When ignorance or denial exists in your mind, there is no room to educate yourself, and the universe has no choice but to bring you another opportunity to humble yourself, create space, and learn. *However, when you align with truth, creation accelerates.*

This works the exact same way in relationships, sports performance, business, and spiritual growth. The more aligned you are with the truth of "what is"—the undeniable facts and reality of the situation at hand—the less effort your ego must expend, because there is less conflict with whatever truth is in front of you. This allows you to more efficiently achieve the success you desire. In this highly locked-in state, you operate like a Zen master or a true sage. You are so in tune with truth that you see how things are coming together before they happen and therefore you masterfully stay ahead of the curve with your choices.

Ignorance leads to suffering and destruction; awareness leads to peace and accelerated creation.

The path of awareness and the ability to adjust to an evolving and changing world are keys to an enlightened way of life. Therefore, I urge you to choose your "I AM"s carefully. Any resistance to your current circumstances indicates conflict and potentially a lot of frustration and prolonged disharmony ahead. The optimal way to begin to change these conflicts is by first acknowledging and accepting what *is* in the world.

OWNING YOUR NARRATIVE AND STORY

The power of self-awareness lies in the knowledge of how you are directing your identity. Many people simply do not realize the power of their narrative and words. *The way you speak reveals what you believe to be true about yourself.* For example, when you do something in error, you may say, "I AM so stupid." This may seem like a casual comment when you say it, but it is revealing a driving truth in your subconscious mind that has a very limiting effect on your reality.

Next-level mindfulness includes being hyperaware of the language you use and how you speak of yourself.

> "Do not speak bad of yourself for the warrior within you hears those words and is lessened by them."
>
> —Samurai proverb

Self-limiting statements that begin with the phrase "I AM" or stray thoughts like "I can't do that," "I won't ever be able to do that," or "I AM always messing that up" limit your creative ability. Even more importantly, limiting statements are *not true*. This is a very pointed example of how manipulative the ego can be when it wants to hold you back from expansive change.

A major step in the process of harnessing the power of "I AM" is to become aware of the self-defining statements or "I AM" statements that have worked against you. How many things can you think of right now that you have talked yourself out of attempting to learn or convinced yourself that you can't do? *Can't* is not true. Do not use this word when describing yourself and your ability. It limits the truth of infinite possibility. The truth, until it changes, is "I have not *been able to do that . . . yet.*" If your intent is to empower yourself and live from an invincible mindset, change the limiting wording "I won't ever be able to do that" to *"I will do that"* or *"I can do this"* or *"I AM doing this."*

The statement "I AM always messing that up" is false and limiting because the word *always* indicates the past, present, and future. The statement is only one-third true. "I *have* messed that up" uses the proper tense and expresses the truth. Anything can happen in this moment and nobody knows what the future holds, making the statement with the word *always* false. The future is a sacred mystery full of infinite possibilities that must be respected while you prepare and plan for it.

The intent behind being hyperaware of how you speak about yourself is to realign your truth in a way that serves your desires. This shifts the expression of your energy so that it aligns with exactly what you want. This shift is the basis for constructing a new reality.

This new reality originates from a narrative of new "I AM" statements: "I AM capable of experiencing that," "I AM worthy enough to experience that," and "I AM smart and studious enough to accomplish that." These are powerful supporting "I AM" statements. The more you take control over how you think and feel, the more life meets you with experiences that harmonize with these declarations.

The difference this shift can make in your life can be likened to driving a boat in the ocean. If you do not take conscious control over how you think and feel about who you are, it is like having a weak motor or sputtering engine that has trouble propelling you to your destination. The wind and the waves in the water around you will overpower your boat and carry you to places you don't really want to go. You will be affected by the energy and wake of every other boat. You'll have little engine power and will end up being pushed around by the currents in your surroundings.

With a strong sense of identity and a strong will and belief, you'll have a powerful engine that can cut through any of life's headwinds and waves. Nothing will be able to knock you off course! You'll speed faster to your dreams and desired destinations.

LIFE'S DIVINE CONNECTION TO YOU

One of the most exciting and secret understandings about life is that everything outside your mind is interacting with you and being drawn into your reality by way of your truth expressed as "I AM."

It is not just how you define yourself or the actions you take that create your reality. In the most beautiful and elegant co-creative process, life meets you with the necessary conditions or learning experiences to help you complete the experience of your self-defining truths. Life knows exactly what you believe to be true. *What a revelation of the power that is in your hands!*

I had the following conversation with a client about embracing a new declared identity:

CLIENT: So I say "I AM" and then something positive after it?

ME: Yes, but the power in the statement is not just saying "I AM," but genuinely believing it to be true.

CLIENT: What if I don't believe it?

ME: Well, you can't fool the universe. It will be a spiritually empty or dead behavior. You'll be going through the motions of announcing new things about yourself, but very little will likely change. Your actions will lack authenticity, and life will also mirror this attitude back with limited results.

CLIENT: How do I truly say it and believe it to the point where it actually has power?

ME: By doing the exact work you're doing now on self-awareness, self-love, and opening to the truth of new possibilities. *By seeing your undeniable worth.* This is what authentically fuels the declaration. This and removing any thoughts that run counter to the new truth you are embracing. Inspired actions that fulfill those "I AM"s are what should automatically come next.

CLIENT: How long do I need to remind myself of these statements?

ME: Until you embody them without prompts or reminders. Until they are ingrained into every fiber of your being without you having to even think about it.

One of life's greatest gifts to you is your ability to define, declare, and demonstrate who you choose to be.

The creative process all starts with intention. What do you want to experience? What do you want to accomplish? What energy and impact do you want to have each day of your life? The world is yours in terms of possibilities. You now know you are worthy and deserving of your dreams, so the only question is: What does it look like and feel like when you dream it?

SETTING YOUR INTERNAL GPS

One of the best exercises I ever learned for manifesting was the process of goal setting. I figured out how to set the GPS for the direction of my entire life by writing down a list of very specific goals. So many people have ideas about what they want or desire, but often these are just fleeting thoughts or wishes in their heads. There is a way to organize and focus these intentions. When you consecrate your goals by putting them on paper, something magical happens. When you take the time to crystalize your vision in words on paper, you amplify the power behind your intentions. By way of its divine awareness and connection to you, life seems to take more notice of your written intended desires

In 1991 I was a year and a half out of college. I had student loan debt, was looking to make more money at my job, and was living with a friend in a two-bedroom apartment. Always trying to learn more, I read a few self-improvement books. Many had the common theme of setting goals. So I decided to take this advice to heart and try it out. One afternoon I simply closed my bedroom door, sat at my desk with a pen and paper, and for the next several hours wrote down everything I could think of that I wanted to accomplish in my entire life. It was a lengthy list that spanned the next sixty or so years. I opened my mind as much as I could to what I wanted my life to look like at each time period and then set it to paper. The process started slowly, but as I wrote one thing down, another vision popped up. I kept imagining what I wanted and writing down what really resonated with me. I had no idea what I was creating by having the faith to put a sincere effort into this process. Before long, my creative intention was effortlessly flowing.

When I finished the list, I read it all, looked at it, and shook my head. These were big things for me at the time. I smiled at the thought of accomplishing even a small portion of this list, given where I was at this moment in my life. I then took a deep breath, folded the list up, put it away in a safe place, and went on with my day.

Twenty years later, I was cleaning out a box of personal things in my home office when I stumbled upon the list. I remember freezing upon seeing it at the bottom of a box. I knew exactly what it was. I carefully picked it up, slowly opened the four tightly folded pages of yellow legal paper, and began to read. My jaw hit the floor. I could not believe the number of goals on the list that I'd actually already achieved!

When I'd written these things down twenty years ago, I'd had absolutely no idea how they would come into being. Not a clue. Yet here I was reading this list and checking off about 80 percent of what I'd written down and wanted to accomplish by this stage of my life. A few of the major things that I'd wanted to experience later in my life had actually come earlier! The job I wanted to get. The woman I wanted to meet. The skill level at golf I wanted to achieve. The certain car I wanted to buy. The house I wanted to live in. The area I wanted to live in. The trips I wanted to take. The income levels I wanted to begin to achieve. The children I wanted to have! It went on and on and on. Truly, I was flabbergasted.

There were some things on the list that I had not achieved, but candidly, over time, my interest in or intent on these things had faded a bit. There were many other things that I had not accomplished yet that were still a work in progress. But holy cow, was I glad I'd taken this seriously and taken the time to do this exercise with intent and care.

The following is the exact exercise I did over thirty-five years ago. I strongly urge you to harness the power of your intentions and do this exercise for yourself now. It does not matter what age you are or where you are in your life at this point. The power behind this exercise in this moment is the same.

LIFE GOAL MAPPING EXERCISE

Choose a time and a place where you will not be distracted and can be completely focused until you finish the exercise. I would set aside a minimum of two undisturbed hours. Prepare the room with decent lighting; an uncluttered, clean space on a table or desk on which to write; and a comfortable chair. Also take measures to ensure your mind is clear, balanced, and relaxed. When you're ready, take the following steps:

1. Title the paper "My Life Goals."

2. Date the paper. It is intended to be a living document that can be amended or updated. I didn't amend mine for twenty years, but it can be updated every year, in five years, or really whenever you want.

3. Create ten sections, leaving a decent amount of space between each. Title the sections as follows:
   - "By Tomorrow"
   - "In One Month"
   - "In Three Months"
   - "In Six Months"

- "In One Year"
- "In One to Three Years"
- "In Three to Five Years"
- "In Five to Ten Years"
- "In Ten to Twenty-Five Years"
- "Within This Lifetime"

4. Go to the first section, close your eyes, take a few deep breaths, and ask yourself what you really want to accomplish or experience in that time frame. Then, without hesitation, begin to write. Do not worry if nothing comes to mind at first. Keep the pen near the paper and when you get a vision, a feeling, or a thought, write it down. Write as many goals as you can, starting with "I AM." Keep writing until you feel you have truly exhausted what you want to accomplish in that time frame.

   Let your mind open to the biggest possibilities and the most desired outcomes. In other words, *dream big*. This is the time to stretch the boundaries of your belief in what is possible for you.

5. No matter what you write, no matter how big you dream, *do not judge what you write*. Do not judge

what you desire, do not scoff at it, do not limit it, and do not edit it in any way to make it more "realistic." After you've written it, believe it and leave it! Then go to the next time frame section and repeat the process.

6. When you have completed all the sections, read the entire list and embrace every outcome, see every vision, and feel every emotion. At the end of reading the list, simply say, "And so it is . . ."

7. Put the list in an envelope and tuck it away in a safe place. Live your life, and let it be. You can read it, revisit it, and add to it any time you like. Just remember to revise it with the same deliberate care you used when creating it. This is important because it demonstrates your intention and your true belief in the creative process of life.

You do not have to know how the goals you listed will be accomplished. Also, the perceived or so-called odds of what you want happening are irrelevant when it comes to the power of creation. Just stay in the place of intention and consistent action and adjustment toward these visions.

> "Even if you can't just snap your fingers and
> make a dream come true, you can travel in
> the direction of your dream, every single day,
> and you can shorten the distance between the
> two of you."
>
> —Douglas Pagels

THE UNIVERSE KNOWS YOUR INTENTIONS

Intentions that are born out of your "I AM" statements are like seeds that can sprout at any moment. Every true wish and desire you declare is known and remembered by life. If what you want hasn't come together for you, know that this is only because the necessary conditions have not yet been met. Rest assured, the universe will deliver to you either the awareness or the tangible conditions you need to accomplish your intent. This delivery could show up as certain people, places, experiences, lessons, or challenges, or as knowledge and awareness, like what is coming to you at this moment from the pages of this book.

An interesting personal example of how the universe keeps a log of your highest intentions takes me back to when I had just turned fifteen years old. Like I often did, I was watching golf on TV with my grandfather. He introduced me to the game and I instantly fell in love with it. We often played together and watched the tournaments on TV. The event we were watching was the 1982 US Open at

Pebble Beach, where Tom Watson famously chipped in for a birdie in dramatic fashion on the seventeenth hole to beat Jack Nicklaus to win. I was glued to the action as I watched him win and hold up the beautiful and legendary US Open trophy with the stunning background of the Pacific Ocean behind him. It was then that I turned to my grandfather and said, "Gramps, I AM going to be holding up that trophy someday!" My grandfather just chuckled. However, in my mind I was as certain about this as I could be. While I played a lot of golf in my teens, twenties, and thirties, I was nowhere close to a professional level of play. I was dedicated and played decently as a mid-single-digit handicap, but that was about as good as it was going to get based on my intent.

Twenty-four years later, in the summer of 2006, I was invited by a member of a prestigious private country club in Arizona to play a round of golf. This is a private club that happens to have many PGA Tour players as members. After our round, we had a late bite to eat in the clubhouse, and as we were on our way out, we passed by the huge trophy case in the men's locker room. One trophy in the very back of the case caught my eye. It was the US Open trophy.

The United States Golf Association (USGA) awards the trophy to the winner of the US Open right after the event and the winner gets to keep it for one year. After that, the winner must return the original trophy to the USGA and in turn they get a replica that they can keep. That year Geoff Ogilvy had won the US Open at Winged Foot Golf Club. Since he was a member of the private club I was playing at that day, he kept it in the club's trophy case for, ahem, safe-keeping. The timing couldn't have been better.

I immediately pulled my flip phone out of my pocket to take a picture of it. Just at the moment I was about to snap the picture, the young locker-room attendant, the only one besides us who was left in the entire club that late in the afternoon, came running up with a key to the case and said, "Hold on a second." I prepared for him to open the case so I could take a picture without getting the glare from the glass. He proceeded to open the case, reach in the back, and grab the trophy. At this point an image flashed in my mind of the US Golf Association police coming around the corner to arrest us. I was certain no one was supposed to touch that trophy. Nonetheless, this young man grabbed the trophy, handed it to me, and said, "Here, you hold the trophy, and I'll take a picture of you holding it up." I looked at my friend to my left and then looked to my right as if to make sure we weren't going to get in trouble, held up the trophy like I had just fought for four days through the toughest conditions in golf to win the US Open, and smiled ear to ear as the attendant took the photo. It was a very fun moment.

As I held it up, I looked at the names inscribed all over the trophy. Ben Hogan, Sam Snead, Byron Nelson, Arnold Palmer, Jack Nicklaus, Lee Trevino, Payne Stewart, Tom Watson, Tiger Woods—I was mesmerized. I could feel the energy in this incredible piece of history as I imagined it sitting on the fireplace mantle or in the trophy case of so many of the greatest golfers of all time.

At thirty-nine years old, I felt like a little kid. When I got home, my wife saw the smile on my face and said, "You must have played well." I said, "No, not exactly, but I did get to hold the US Open trophy!" "Wow," she said, "that's great! How did that happen?" As I proceeded to tell her all about it, a memory floated into the forefront of my mind about that time when I was a kid watching the 1982 US Open with my grandfather and dreaming one day of this moment. Now here that moment was. I did it.

Then it hit me.

"Oh nooo!" I shouted. "What's wrong?" my wife said with a concerned look. Exasperated, I looked at her and said, "When I was a kid and was watching the US Open on TV with my grandfather, I told him, 'One day that is going to be me. I AM going to hold that US Open trophy up.' Why didn't I say, 'One day that's going to be me. I AM going to *win* the US Open'?"

The moral of the story is to be very exact with your intentions. The universe listens and does not forget. I said that it was going to be me "holding" the trophy someday. When the conditions were right, the universe delivered perfectly on this declaration. A more mindful me would have been much more specific regarding the statement. Oh well, next lifetime.

The exact sequence of events that had to occur to make the self-declaration I made at a young age come true is pretty interesting. I had to be asked to play at that particular golf club. We had to be the last ones in the clubhouse or else I'm certain that attendant would not have opened that locked case. I had to notice the trophy in the back of the case out of the corner of my eye. Ogilvy had to be a member and keep his trophy at the club. And most astonishingly, the young locker-room attendant had to hear me as I spoke about the trophy and think, *I'll get the keys, open the case for the guy, hand him the trophy, and take a picture of him holding it.* Really?

My point is that none of this is by chance. The universe knows your intentions and knows exactly what pieces need to move into place to accomplish those intentions. Your job is to just keep doing your part to demonstrate your desires and intentions. Life will use the right people and circumstances to increase the probability of your intentions occurring. Now, here's where it gets a little more interesting. When I was a kid, I made a statement I truly believed could happen. That belief never changed. I may have known in my late teens that being a professional golfer was not my career path, but the thought of not holding the trophy never crossed my mind. *The thought was still alive with energy as an intention and belief out in the ether of the universe.* When the conditions were right, it germinated and manifested.

It's the same when it comes to your day-to-day life. You never know when the moment of manifestation will come. You must simply keep the intention strong, stay optimistic, and trust where your intuition and heart take you. Whether it's in business, sports, or relationships, you must keep your mind open to any possibility. This is the key to keeping the conditions moving in favor of your dreams materializing. So be exact in your vision and stay ready. It tends to happen when you least expect it!

The self-defining power of "I AM" and the power of putting your intentions down on paper were demonstrated at the highest level when I was working in Major League Baseball for the Tampa Bay Rays in 2016. I started my work with the Rays by giving a speech on the power of mindfulness and mental strength to the entire team in spring training. During a couple of spring training games, several players approached me in the dugout and expressed an interest in learning more and taking this work further to advance their mindset and mental approach. One of these players was three-time All-Star, two-time Gold Glove Award winner, and team leader Evan Longoria. While I was not surprised that many of the younger guys on the team were really interested in this work, I was pleasantly surprised when veteran and team star "Longo" sat down next to me in the dugout, slapped my thigh, and said, "I want to learn more about your work." We started working together immediately.

What makes great athletes or people who achieve extraordinary things so amazing is not only their incredible work ethic but their open and curious minds. Here was a top MLB player who had been playing successfully in the big show for eight years and was still looking to learn, grow, and continue to push the boundaries of his performance. He had no resistance or hesitation, just a raw hunger to always be the best he could be, using all the resources life presented him to help in that effort. I was honored to be a small part of that journey.

During our first meeting in spring training, we pulled two folding chairs into a broom closet for privacy. Yes, these were the early days of teams using mental strength training! In that meeting, one of the questions I asked Longo was if he'd ever focused on setting goals or written down any self-defining statements. He said no and explained that he had a journal in his locker that someone bought for him a few years ago, but he only used it for fantasy football notes. I told him to go grab it.

One of the first things I had him do, using the new mentality of infinite possibilities we worked on, was to write down some new goals and intentions for his desired performance in the form of "I AM" statements. The key was that he had to make sure the goals were big enough to make him more than a little uncomfortable. They had to be things he hadn't accomplished before in his career. These were things that would stretch his identity as a player to another level. He understood completely and wrote down his intentions for some key offensive production numbers he wanted to accomplish for the entire season.

That year Evan Longoria hit more home runs than he'd ever hit before in a single season. Thirty-six times he "went yard." At thirty years of age, he had one of the best offensive years of his amazing career. Taking desire, talent, curiosity, hunger, and humility and combining it with the wisdom of infinite potential is a potent recipe for success. Longoria did not let any past limitations or preconceived notions of possibility affect who he could be. He then brought this vision into his mindset and daily approach. He opened the doors of his mind to let a lifetime of experience and talent shine freely to create even more possibility for himself.

STAY OPEN TO NEW ANSWERS

The co-creative relationship with life is a very exact process. The minute you set an intention with the statement "I AM," life begins its astonishing process of creation. A million things are beginning to line up for you below the surface of reality. Just like the seed germinating and growing in the darkness underground with no signs of growth on the surface, the momentum of your efforts can seem hidden. At times it can seem like your intentions and desires are not taking root or showing any movement or momentum. Do not get discouraged! This is where trust in the process is imperative. If you keep moving toward what you want and you keep learning and nurturing the process, eventually you'll see your desired outcome begin to materialize.

What's interesting about the creative process is that most people believe that it is their thoughts, choices, and actions that create their reality. While this is a big part of how it works, the truly magical and mystical part is how the universe responds to your will. All of the life around you knows exactly what you are trying to create and is working in harmony with you. You might ask, "Well, why hasn't what I've wanted materialized yet?" The simple and exact answer is that the necessary conditions are not in place either internally in your awareness or externally in the conditions around you. Your next logical question would be, "What conditions are missing?" Now we are getting somewhere, because many people are simply not ready to either ask this question or face the reasons why what they want hasn't happened yet. They want to blame it on anything else. This is not the path of mastery. The path to success is about taking full responsibility not only for the actions you take but also for learning what it takes to become who you want to be. When it comes to any quest, as the Rolling Stones song says, "you can't always get what you want, but if you try sometimes, you might just find, you get what you need."

These "answers" are available to you every day. What controls the speed of both the delivery of these answers and your ability to see them and embrace them is the level of your will for change. *It is not until your faith is 1 percent stronger than your fear that change and transformation can occur.* This is when you will expand your comfort zone and open up to a new way of life. You are pacing your experience of time.

The following list may seem simple, but the entries represent everyday examples of the options that can immediately create change and move you closer to what you say you want.

At any moment you can decide to:

- have the hard conversation with your significant other.
- create your résumé and send it out to job prospects.

- take your athletic talent to the next level with grit and a new open mindset.
- read the book on spirituality slowly, deeply, and meaningfully.
- enter rehab and truly commit to the full recovery process.
- go on the date or the dating app with optimism and hope.
- call and reconcile with your family member.
- decide to finally be vulnerable and commit to consistent honesty.
- reflect on your past negativity and self-centeredness and commit to being a new person.
- write your creed and dedicate yourself to who you now want to be.
- finally take on the responsibility of being healthy.

Each of these choices are designed to put a "wrinkle in the pattern" of your previous behavior by demonstrating a new intention. This is the definition of transformation. A new version of your soul is being born. It may feel a little scary and a little unfamiliar as you step into an unknown experience, but this is exactly how you stretch your awareness and create yourself anew.

When you make this internal shift, you will see a change in how others treat you. This means that the frequency of your energy will dictate a new aura and state of being. Since reality is one infinite process of creation, everything in existence is supporting everything else toward that creation. So basically, the people in your life are serving your beliefs. When you authentically change how you declare and demonstrate who you are, the individuals around you will change and switch to begin to serve your new beliefs and the new version of you.

Here are a few subtle and common examples of how your reality can dramatically improve over time when there is a consistent positive change in how you see yourself ("I AM").

At work:

- A boss may treat you better and pay you more money.
- A client may give you some great referrals.
- A big order may come your way.
- A great promotion or job opportunity may present itself.

In sports:

- A coach may acknowledge you and give you more playing time and attention.
- Your teammates may look to you for confidence and leadership.
- The game may slow down and you may find yourself mentally and physically in complete control of what's happening.
- You may start winning more, making more shots, burying more putts, executing in more at bats, and

playing more freely, more confidently, and with more focus.

In relationships:

- A significant other may treat you in a more loving and respectful way.
- Love may flow more abundantly in your life.
- Opportunities to meet people and go out may increase.
- Your relationship may shift and become more joyful.

In other areas of life:

- People may open doors for you and cars may stop to let you in on the road.
- Your work, art, or craft may suddenly become more recognized.
- Help in certain areas of your life may show up more serendipitously.
- An investment may suddenly work out in a big way.
- Your health may dramatically improve.

You enter the flow of life when you are more aware of how it all works. This occurs when you are in harmony with creation and the process of creation. There will always be lessons in life, but with less resistance to and ignorance of how life truly works, your ability to manifest elevates.

Hence, you become a master of your reality in a way that puts you in the zone, not just in one area of life but in all areas of your life.

The invincible mind is an incredibly sacred state of being. A place where intuition flourishes and life bends to your will. In this state you have realized your power as a creator and are open to the beauty of life and where it takes you in terms of your peak potential. Your dreams are now closer than you may have ever imagined. A new you is now emerging.

When you are creating a new you, new "I AM" statements are a very effective way to set these changes deep into your identity. However, as life-changing as new "I AM" statements are, they have no creative power without your authentic belief supporting each of them. The process can't be faked. It's like having a bottle with a magical genie in it. You can rub the bottle all you want, but the genie will not come out to grant your wishes until your heart is pure with a belief in the genie's power.

The following is a very important and powerful list of personal declarations. Each is an "I AM" statement that encapsulates the learnings in the first six steps of this book. I recommend that you read these out loud to yourself until each statement can be embraced deeply into your soul. When you are in complete harmony with these statements, you should have no discomfort in reading them out loud. Do this as many times as you need to, until the deepest part of you feels the comfort, peace, and power that come with these statements.

- I AM grateful for this sacred eternal moment.
- I AM a perfect creation born of a perfect universe.
- I AM here now as matter because I matter.
- I AM exactly where I'm supposed to be at this moment on my creative journey.
- I AM aware of the infinite possibilities that are always available to me.
- I AM worthy of what I imagine and dream of for myself.
- I AM aware of how I co-create with life.
- I AM committed to learning every day.
- I AM faithful that each day has purpose for me.
- I AM capable of anything I put my mind to and am willing to work toward.
- I AM mindful of my divine connection to all of life.
- I AM respectful of my ability to express myself as I choose and of others' ability to do the same.
- I AM conscious of my power to love myself unconditionally and my power to demonstrate that unconditional love to others.
- I AM who I choose to be now!

Free

What a quest to be free.
Still absorbing it's real.
A door to a new life,
These beautiful vibes I now feel.

Who knew the key
Was always close by.
A misunderstanding of self,
I can no longer lie.

The truth is right here.
I'm love's incarnation.
Art without flaw.
Life's divine presentation.

My future now hopeful,
My soul now clean.
I've finally met myself.
For the first time, I'm me.

This changes everything,
The simple grace of this state.
My mind now on creation.
Unlimited becomes my fate.

Time to focus on love.
Infinite choices now beckon.
Free reign of mind.
A million lifetimes to reckon!

PART THREE

NEXT-LEVEL

MINDFULNESS

MASTERING CHALLENGES AND NEGATIVITY

How to Conquer the Tests and Traps of Life

Every storm runs out of rain.

—Maya Angelou

As you go forward creating your intentions from a more mindful and empowered state, life may confront you with some minor and major challenges, tests, and traps along the way. The invincible mind is ready for any of them. Remember, life will constantly look to validate that you are who you say you are. The more prepared you are to respond in a masterful way, the more effortlessly your life will flow.

TRUSTING THERE IS PURPOSE IN CHALLENGES

The synchronicity and elegance of life are found in how it meets you in the process of endless creation. Life will use every experience to move you closer to your intentions. This includes negative and challenging experiences. The mindset of infinite possibilities and inevitable success requires you to be ready for these experiences should they happen, and be trusting that each of these experiences are happening for a specific reason. The more prepared you are, the less any of these situations, if they arise, will shock you or disrupt your mental clarity and balance.

An invincible mind is able to see both order and opportunity in any seeming chaos. Will there be surprise? Yes. Will there be grief? Yes. Will there be moments of fear as things suddenly shift or change in your reality without much warning? Yes. But it will be the way you respond to these tests and challenges that will make all the difference in what happens next. Your reactions will determine what you still have to learn and how much suffering and time will play a role in these lessons. Genuine, grounded faith in all you have learned about the bigger picture of how life works will be imperative as you process these events.

If you have a setback, encounter a sudden change to your plans, or life throws you a major curveball, take a breath and remind yourself that there is something in this for you. *There are no wasted moments in life.* Every small detail you experience is part of the perfection of the conditions coming together for whatever it is you are moving toward creating, or whatever awareness is required for you to learn. By "perfect," I mean not "optimal" but "exact." A perfect sequence of previous events has brought whatever the current challenge, delay, obstacle, or circumstance is into your life.

Arguing with what already exists or happened in the past is a futile endeavor. I say this not to seem cold or show a lack of empathy for your situation, but to guide you on the path to mental mastery over any challenges or sudden changes in your reality. This knowledge is here to help you stay as balanced as possible, and if you do happen to get thrown off by your circumstances, even just a bit, this information is here to help move you back into a state of empowerment quickly and with as little suffering as possible.

Grief is normal and natural. When change occurs, it is healthy to grieve the change and the loss. This could be the loss of a great job, a sports defeat, the end of a loving relationship, or even the sudden passing of a loved one. There are no rules on how long one should grieve. This is a very personal process. However, there is a message for you in all that enters and exits your reality.

Furthermore, the wisdom you acquire as you overcome difficulties and develop the skills to master future events is necessary not only for your own well-being but also for the benefit of many of the people around you. Part of the purpose of any difficult experience is for you to share the perspective and wisdom you've gained in order to help other people in their time of difficulty.

The invincible mindset really all comes down to trust. You must come to trust that while there are things we all must go through that cause pain and suffering, there is nothing that this divine universe brings into your existence that is without purpose. Sometimes you'll connect the dots right away, and other times you may have to wait years until the time is right for you to understand why something had to occur in a certain way. But rest assured, this time does come. The acceptance of this idea is the essence of faith.

The loss of my mother was one of the most difficult experiences I have ever gone through. It was sudden and unexpected. The void is unfillable, and the love lost is irreplaceable. However, because I have learned to trust life, as painful as the absence of my mother feels to me, I know that there is something profound for me to understand in this very difficult experience. I also have faith that what I've been through will in some way help others who will go through similar situations.

Life often does not give us the lesson we want when teaching us, because who would ever choose such a lesson? We get our lessons when life, God, or the universe deems it to be *the right time* for that particular lesson. Experiencing loss is an unavoidable destiny for each of us and is simply a part of life. When these things happen, we become more appreciative of all of creation because we realize its fragile and finite nature. Therefore, we gain the wisdom and grace that only real-life experiences of loss can provide.

Every single human being has a different life to live and a

different path to travel for how this type of lesson of loss unfolds in their lifetime. Some people experience these harsh lessons early in life and some later. However, everyone has similar lessons to learn and the same trust and faith to develop. Each person is simply at a different point on the infinite unfolding spiral of consciousness we all are traveling.

MASTERING THE CHALLENGES AND TESTS ON YOUR PATH

You are always connected to the universe. How could the cosmos, which birthed you into existence and ushered you to this very moment, ever leave you without access to insight? It never has, and it never will. Your relationship with creativity or divinity is inescapable. Included in this relationship are the unavoidable learnings and growth process you must go through to evolve and survive as intended or desired.

At this point in your process of learning the invincible mindset, it is empowering to contemplate the following questions:

How can I be prepared for any possibility in a way that keeps me in full control of my mindset?

How can I reduce fear, anxiety, and suffering when I am in the midst of a learning experience?

How can I use the knowledge I've gained from past challenges and tests to overcome my current situation?

How can I turn and face any future challenges with a Zen-like perspective?

How can I use my understanding of self-definition to express who I desire to be right now?

How can I use the wisdom I've learned from what I have already been through to help another who is struggling?

Each of these questions has answers that can be found more efficiently when you face any personal challenge and deal with any fear or uncertainty head-on. Rather than avoiding what may seem like a difficult learning opportunity, it is most beneficial to take the time to slow down and see and embrace what life is trying to teach you.

> "God wants us to walk, but the devil sends a
> limo."
>
> —Val Kilmer

Avoiding life's tough lessons will bring you no closer to having, doing, or being what you want. In fact, avoiding what a tough lesson or situation is trying to teach you will do just the opposite: it will create more of what you do not want to experience. While short-term avoidance may prevent you from having to face your fears or deal with the reality of an uncomfortable truth, it will only add to the karma of what you will have to learn and go through in the future. The universe will continue to teach the same lessons you tried to escape in a new situation. It's like the universe is saying to you, "We can do this the easy way, or we can do this the hard way. It's your choice." Grounding yourself in the unshakable trust that life is working with you regardless of how your path is unfolding can provide an immediate sense of calm. It can also turn confusion and resistance into a search for insight and wisdom.

When you want to get to the next level in a video game, you can't skip mastering the level you're on. Similarly, when you want to accelerate your path to fulfillment, you can't avoid tough lessons of humility. Instead, contemplate what life is offering you and trying to tell you in every challenge you face. There you will find the key to leveling up.

Flip Your Perspective

When you want to increase your creative power, shifting the perspective from "Why is this happening to me?" to "What do I have to learn or gain by what is happening to me?" is a masterful way to do it. Another powerful shift is to change your perspective from feeling like it's all happening *to you* to feeling like it is all happening *for you* in some way.

In my work with some of the top athletes in the world on mental performance, one of the most effective techniques I've taught them for facing adversity is to take on a different angle of attack when responding to a difficult situation. Any time they are not performing up to their true potential, I tell them that instead of getting frustrated or angry at themselves, they should get inquisitive. In other words, do not stay in resistance and emotion, *use the challenge to see what life is offering you!*

Anger is resistance. So, while a disappointment can cause an initial outburst of emotion, which is normal for any athlete, beyond that moment of release, the experience is about gathering information and learning. The athlete should ask, "What has caused this to happen? How can I change this going forward? What can I learn from this?" This works for any tough situation you face, whether or not you're an athlete.

I remember watching the New England Patriots quarterback Tom Brady in the conference championship playoff game in 2012 when the Patriots were playing the Ravens. There were two minutes to go on the clock, and the Patriots had the ball on their own thirty-yard line. Of course, everyone thought Brady was going to lead them down the field to victory. This was a rare occasion when he did not. He threw an interception with a minute to go in the game. The Ravens then ran the clock out and sealed the victory.

The interesting part was after Brady threw the interception and the TV camera showed him back on the sideline. The game and the season were basically over, but what was Brady doing? Was he pouting and brooding? Was he yelling at teammates? Was he standing around waiting to head to the locker room or thinking about vacation? No, he was sitting on the bench, his head buried in his computer tablet, reviewing the previous play and trying to figure out what he'd missed and what had gone wrong. He was trying to learn from it! Not for the current season, which was over, but for the many seasons and new opportunities he knew would come. Tom Brady did not waste any opportunity to get better. This seemingly insignificant moment on the sideline revealed his faith and focus on the bigger picture. The knowledge he gained in this moment may well have been used *in any one of his five future Super Bowl victories!* This bigger vision and the faith to seize all of life's learning opportunities are essential attributes of an invincible mind.

The best athletes and the most successful people in any field are extremely curious about what they need to learn to continue to execute at the highest level possible. They don't waste their time resisting what's happening or blaming someone else. They take advantage of the moment and the information that life presents them, and they make adjustments until they get it right.

Nolan Ryan, arguably the greatest pitcher in Major League Baseball history, said it best about the mental challenges of baseball in an interview by Tim Wendel titled "Nolan Ryan's Secret to Success." Ryan, who played for twenty-nine years, threw a record seven career no-hitters, and still holds the record for the most strikeouts in MLB history with 5,714, said, "I've learned if you can't handle the mental side of it, you're never going to be able to handle the physical side of it." He added, "When you get to the top level, there's not a lot of separation in the physical abilities of players. It's the mental approach to the game that separates people."

Having the mental strength to face challenges head-on is a courageous and empowered way to go through any area of life. When you're ready to step up, the optimal question to ask is, "What is in this challenge that will help get me to where I want to go?" Like a scientist, you are looking for the right combination of ingredients to complete the formula.

Yes, you will go through times of struggle and learning. But does the champion on any battlefield have no scars? Has the individual who finds true love not lived through previous heartbreak? Isn't the successful entrepreneur someone who has risked and lost—perhaps staking and losing every dime they had multiple times—before finally getting their business model right?

Tests and challenges in your life are meant to help strengthen your mind, sharpen your blade, and increase your competence. These moments build resiliency and grit, which prepares you for the bigger challenges and victories yet to come.

"A smooth sea never made a skilled sailor."
—Franklin D. Roosevelt

Find the Silver Lining

Learning to mine a silver lining or to redeem something from tough situations is a very powerful way of navigating deep traumas and tragedies. Mine every experience you can for its hidden treasure, and you will soar through the process of learning. As painful as life can seem at times, there is always a priceless gem of wisdom to be found that will prove invaluable someday.

Here are a few silver linings you can dig for when faced with tough situations in your life. You get to:

- learn why it's happening and what's in it for you.
- show your strength of will and your fortitude to go on.
- define who you are and inspire others through your resiliency and response.
- develop wisdom through experience.
- know the grace of handling or overcoming any difficult situation.
- practice shifting your perspective to gratitude.

The Importance of Gratitude

To help you through any tough situation that challenges your beliefs or puts you in a vulnerable state of anxiety, one major tool is gratitude. Gratitude is what allows you to rebalance your state of mind, moving you from a place of fear, lack, and worry *to a place of perspective on what you do have.* When things don't go as expected or planned, your ego tends to focus on what you don't have or what has been taken away from you. It is imperative at these times of imbalance to go to a place of perspective by focusing on something that is good, or what you do have in your life, or what you still can do.

For example, do you have a roof over your head? Do you have people who care about you and love you? Do you have food? Do you have access to clean water? Are you alive and able to breathe? Remember to use the truth and perspective of gratitude to keep you in a mindful, clear, and respectful state no matter what you are going through.

THE POWER OF PERSEVERANCE: DESTINY'S STORY

Some years ago, I was a keynote speaker at a retreat for a big company with products that empower employees to build their own business from home. In one of the breakout sessions I hosted, I was discussing major life challenges and how to overcome them. Toward the end of the session, when I was talking about the power of trust and faith, a petite young woman stood up in the back of the room and said, "I know about overcoming challenge and having faith." Then she started to tell her story. It is one of the most powerful examples of perseverance, trust, and faith that I've come across in my work.

Destiny has been through something that would challenge anybody's strength of mind. At fifteen years old, she met her first boyfriend, Corey. They went to school, grew up together, fell in love, and got married when she was eighteen. Three years later, they had a son they named Parker. Their life was starting out as beautifully as they could have hoped. However, just over one year later, life took a tragic turn.

On the way to a work meeting, a drunk driver who was traveling at almost ninety miles an hour crossed the center line of the highway. Destiny and her family, in the car on the other side, were hit head-on. Her precious fifteen-month-old baby boy, Parker, died instantly on impact. Her husband, Corey, who had just turned twenty-two, was airlifted to a nearby hospital, and twenty-four hours later he died as well. The drunk driver was killed instantly. Destiny walked away from the accident with scrapes and bruises and a life that was instantly changed.

From that moment forward, Destiny never stepped foot back in her house. She was heavily medicated after the accident and taken to her mother's home, where she just sat there day after day after day, trying to make sense of the tragic turn her life had taken. Understandably, she felt catatonic. However, after a few weeks something changed. She reached her breaking point. She decided she could no longer just sit there as the days went by. So she started getting up early every day, showering, and just simply going out and driving. She did this for hours on end. On one of those drives, she made the life-changing decision to take her mindset back. She decided that the drunk driver who took so much from her *was not going to take her life from her as well*. So she mustered the trust to go on, and she kept moving forward one day, and often one hour, at a time.

Some days, getting herself out of bed and out for that drive took everything she had, but she did it consistently. When I asked her about it, she said, "I was inspired to keep going so one day I could eventually let the whole world know how precious they are and how precious life is. I wanted my life to be an example that nothing can stop you in life."

Destiny lives in a little town in Missouri where everyone knows everything about everyone else. When she finally started going back out in public, the people she would see all knew her story. They would flock to her, and because they didn't know what else to say or do, they would treat her like a massive charity case. Destiny didn't want that kind of pity or attention, so she stopped going out in public. A couple of months after the accident, she met Brett, a friend of her brother's who had no idea who she was or what she had been through. Finally, she said, "I could talk to someone who didn't know my story or look at me in that tragic light." They continued to talk for months.

In the meantime, Destiny continued to move forward. She went for a drive every day to clear her mind and think. When she did, she promised God that if she ever had the opportunity to have a family again, she would do things differently. She would learn to cherish time more, she would cherish every moment with her loved ones more, and every day she would appreciate the good and trust that there was something to learn in the bad.

Three years after the accident that took so much from Destiny, she married her brother's friend Brett, and they now have two beautiful children: a precious boy named Cohen and a darling little girl named Coraline. They are now living a happy and content life. Destiny truly embodies what it is to have an invincible mindset. Her path is the epitome of using the power of choice to move forward and deal with a seemingly impossible reality.

When she left the retreat where we met, Destiny told me that for the first time in her life, she had learned more about who she is and how truly powerful she really is. Now she knows her ability to love every moment of life and persevere no matter what the challenge. She now knows what she is capable of overcoming and creating. Destiny is also incredibly open about her story and her mission to honor the loss of her son, Parker, and husband, Corey. She is doing so by making sure the world knows about the dangers of drunk or distracted driving. She has become a shining light to so many, and I am beyond honored that I met her and had the chance to work with her, talk to her, and learn from her as well.

MASTERING THE TRAP OF A PROTECTIVE EGO

As you move down the path of infinite potential and possibilities, one of the biggest obstacles you will encounter is your own mind. That's because your ego is designed to protect you from expansion into the unknown.

When you take significant steps to demonstrate a new you, there is likely to be a period of discomfort as you begin. As you stretch the fabric of your soul and become a new version of yourself, your new actions will move you into unfamiliar territory. Your ego will immediately be put on guard. Vulnerability can create fear, and if the new space you are entering makes you fearful or uneasy, your ego will try to pull you back in a number of ways.

Here are some examples of changes that may create fear and send the ego into high alert:

- Starting your first day at a new job with new expectations
- Revealing your art, writing, or music to others for the first time
- Entering a new relationship where you have to become vulnerable
- Making more money than you've ever made before
- Competing in your sport at a new level or with better players for the first time
- Taking on more financial risk to expand your business
- Giving your first speech or giving a speech to a larger than usual group of people
- Moving and starting at a new school or meeting new people

Basically, any time you do something new that expands your identity, you become susceptible to your ego's attempts to pull you back to the original safe and known space. If your ego feels too much is at risk or is uncomfortable with the space, it will do anything to stop you.

In an effort to pull you back to an old comfort zone, the fear-dominated or active ego will tell you that:

- you're not worthy of the job and should quit before you're fired.

- what you created is not good, and no one will want it or care.
- the person you're in a new relationship with is going to use you and leave you once they learn more about you, once you are intimate with them, or once they meet your family.
- you're going to fail or embarrass yourself in a key moment as an athlete.
- you're unworthy of this kind of success or money and you're a fraud.
- your business is going to fail if you take more risks or try to expand
- everyone will laugh at you and your speech
- these new people you're trying to meet will think you are weird and won't like you.

One of the most important things to remember when it comes to the voice in your head is that any negative or limiting statement about you, your ability, your beauty, or your worth is a *lie*.

Do not listen to your ego when it tells you negative or limiting things about who you are.

Your ego can be a massive liar. It lies to you to stop you from creating change when your will or self-belief isn't strong enough yet. Remember these two facts about your ego, and you will take away its power to limit you:

- Your ego will project fear-based outcomes as if they are a certainty to try to stop you from moving forward in your life.
- Your ego does not know the future with any certainty. No one does. There is an infinite number of potential outcomes for your future, including thousands of positive results.

There is no way to avoid being vulnerable if you want to move forward in your life in a new way. The way to master a protective ego and move forward with more ease is to redefine who you are in a way where your ego serves a creative and bold self. For example, you might tell yourself, "I AM capable of achieving this" or, "I AM doing this and will either succeed at it or learn." To do this, you have to push yourself to think and act differently. You quiet the limiting lies of your ego with new, more unlimited thoughts and instructions. The masterful way to live in a space of infinite possibility and to destroy these unhelpful thoughts is to be *aware* of the potential negative limiting and destructive voice of your ego. This will help you be more prepared to immediately counter that limiting voice and redirect your ego with new truth.

When you know you cannot fail in life and that every move forward is a win-win, you are completely empowered. Your awareness, fortitude, and courage strengthen when you remember your perfection and worth. Since the ego's job is to validate personal truth, the stronger any new belief about yourself becomes, the more easily your ego will walk into that new version of yourself, no matter how uncomfortable and vulnerable you've felt. *This is the power of a strong will and belief!* This is how some of the best athletes in the world walk into next-level performance with ease. Their belief is *so* strong that their egos have no choice but to work relentlessly hard to make this truth a reality.

When the voice of the limiting part of your ego shows up, ask yourself these two powerful questions. Write down your answers.

- Is any negative or limiting thought that my mind is trying to tell me about who I am, or what my future will be, true?
- Are these negative and limiting thoughts my mind is telling me helpful to my state of mind and my desire to create what I really want?

The point of these questions is to see if you are in a trap of the ego. The empowered answer to both questions is a resounding no.

Negativity is counter to these encouraging creative states of mind. Change the counterproductive coding and old negative narrative, and redirect your ego. Feed your mind with only the most nurturing, unlimited beliefs possible.

One client I worked with had a tremendous amount of anxiety about being able to make it to the next level in her sport. She was about to take the leap from high school competition to the Division I college level. Her anxiety stemmed from the belief of "not good enough." I helped her look at the core counterproductive belief and challenge it.

ME: Is it true that you are not good enough? You've been recruited because of your outstanding play.

CLIENT: Well, no.

ME: So, where is this belief coming from?

CLIENT: I guess the fear that I will fail.

ME: Have you failed to get to this point in your athletic career?

CLIENT: Well, no...

ME: Do you want to fail?

CLIENT: No.

ME: Has the future happened yet?

CLIENT: No.

ME: No, the future holds infinite possibility. Therefore, any outcome is possible for you, including, let's pick a number, a billion *positive* outcomes. In other words, your ego is lying to you, creating that unnecessary fear. To take back control and strength, let's focus on the positive outcomes that are grounded in the truth of how you got here: your talent, worthiness, and your will and desire!

CLIENT: So, why does the fear feel bigger at times?

ME: Because you feel the stakes are bigger. You feel more vulnerable and outside your comfort zone at this level. There is no difference but the one in your mind. In order to take back control of how you want to feel, you must change your perspective on what's at stake. Your success at this level is important, but to cultivate your strongest state of mind, it can't be everything. You must focus on what *is* possible for you based on your outstanding previous play. You must decide to own the beliefs that support these attainable possibilities and acknowledge that you are just as worthy as anyone else of succeeding at this level! Anything less does not serve you in the highest way.

MASTERING THE TRAP OF GENETIC PULLBACK

One of the most subtle, sneaky, and influential forces on your mindset, perceptions, actions, and reactions is your genes. The genetics you received at conception can have a profound effect on who you are and how your life unfolds. Based on your environment, nurturing, and personal experiences, some of these genes will have more impact on you than others. Some genes' characteristics will be expressed and will become present in your personality and choices. Some of your genes and the characteristics they hold will remain latent and will have no discernible effect on your life. These are genes that have been passed from generation to generation.

The study of how our genes express themselves or change their expression over our lifetime is called epigenetics. The environment you grew up in and the way you were nurtured have a major influence on your genetic expression. What is interesting is that the driver of all genetic change is rooted in what is necessary for survival. If a trait is advantageous and increases the probability for survival, it will be expressed and passed to the next generation.

A big part of self-mastery is being aware of any generational patterns of behavior you want to break.

Generational "curses" are patterns of undesired energy, thought, behavior, physiology, and psychology that repeat in some fashion from one generation to the next. This propensity will live in the genetic coding until a new will for change alters that expression. The expression of these genes can occur naturally or can be triggered by your environment and your nurturing, or these genes can express or materialize as you age. Especially as you get older, how often do you hear yourself talk, laugh, or respond to a comment or a conversation in a way that immediately makes you hear your father's or mother's voice?

Next-level mindfulness is about being acutely aware of any undesired character traits and behaviors so you can change this subtle yet powerful influence over your personality. Being conscious of this deep generational influence or any generational trauma is the pathway to redirecting it and changing its effect on you. Many people are completely unaware of how much their genetics affect their mindset and the quality of their energy. This sneaky force allows undesired traits of your parents or grandparents to emerge at any moment. Expanding and changing your identity, *even if this change is incredibly positive*, can trigger these generational genetic traits. At times these traits can be limiting and destructive. The reason they were originally passed down is that they worked for the previous generation in terms of what was perceived as necessary for survival. However, every generation deals with the world in a different way. Today, we know that your grandfather's or father's use of corporal punishment is not the way to handle discipline. Your grandmother's or mother's use of guilt to manipulate you may not be the instinctual behavior you want to exhibit or pass on to the next generation. Smoking cigarettes to relax like your parents did, as many doctors in the 1950s and '60s promoted, is not the way to achieve health and well-being, as we understand today.

Some of these genetic tendencies or familiar behavior patterns may have been passed on to you. However, to be resilient in your quest for the invincible mindset and take a huge step toward mastery-level awareness, you must be mindful of which behaviors serve you and which ones do not. Next-level mindfulness helps you pause and have enough self-awareness to choose the way you want to define yourself in each moment. It allows you to catch these formerly subconscious tendencies and redirect them. This is how you begin to fundamentally change your nature and identity. *This higher state is how you take command and control over your evolutionary process.*

This subtle trap of genetic pullback is a strong one and will continue until your previously unconscious instincts and behavior patterns have finally been interrupted and changed. You must actively monitor yourself until you don't have to think about your behavior any longer. This is when the switch in the gene for the expression of the old behavior will turn from on to off. It's also equally important to consider how many great traits and positive genetic expressions you received from those who came before you. Remember, regardless of what has unfolded, right here and right now the power is in your hands to define, declare, and demonstrate who you choose to be.

Just because your father used alcohol and drugs to cope does not mean you have to be susceptible to this trap. Just because your mother yelled to get attention and control does not mean you have to demonstrate the same pattern in your life. Just because your grandfather was riddled with physical ailments and debilitating health does not mean you can't take care of yourself differently and live a perfectly healthy and long life. Just because your parents were irresponsible with money doesn't mean you cannot be smart and responsible and reach untold financial success and heights. Just because your parents didn't play sports or didn't reach the level they desired does not mean you can't reach your athletic goals. Just because your mother or father was negative minded and lived in fear and anxiety does not mean you have to carry one ounce of this trait into your life. Just because your parents divorced and had trouble in romantic, loving relationships does not mean you can't have the most amazing, loving relationship at any age.

Over the course of your life, these traits may work their way into your experiences. These traits will flare up especially when you are on a path of expansion and growth. This is because new, grander experiences may represent the opposite of what previous generations were familiar with. The story of the lottery winner who wins millions and ends up in worse financial condition a year later comes to mind. If the lottery winner doesn't develop the value system and financial savvy necessary to maintain their newfound wealth, they will soon find themselves back in the original financial situation or *comfort zone* they were in before winning the money.

This is why it is critical to be aware of the trap of "genetic pullback." These traits can be expressed at any moment. The more aware you are, the more determined you will be to stay unattached to any previous generation's limitations or traits that do not serve you and your desired life.

MASTERING THE TRAP OF NEGATIVE PEOPLE

One of the most influential sources of energy outside your own mind is other people. You can be strongly and subtly affected by the energy of the people you interact with on a daily basis. Family, friends, significant others, coworkers, and influential people in the world can all have a positive or negative impact on your state of energy—*if* you allow it. Mastering the art of deflecting or neutralizing the negative energy of others is a major step toward next-level mindfulness and becoming invincible of mind.

There may be plenty of amazing, supportive, and loving people in your life who lift you up and help you in all that you do. This section is specifically about encounters with those who, for one reason or another, project energy that has a negative effect on you. This is when focus and mindfulness are really important. Like a gymnast on a balance beam, you have to remain focused and committed to staying on your path of positivity rather than allowing yourself to be pulled off into the sea of negativity around you.

When you have an intent to be more limitless or creative, or to live a life filled with more joy and positivity, the people around you will both support you and at times try to hold you back. It is a push-pull relationship. People want to see you do well, as many find joy in your joy, and your actions and experiences inspire them. However, some can also despise the contrast your growth reveals when it makes them feel smaller or "less than." It is not because people are inherently "bad"; it is simply because they are trying to avoid feeling worse than they already feel about themselves, and they don't have the ability to cope with seeing your success.

Stable, happy, content, fulfilled people seem to be a minority in today's world. Therefore, for you to stay on track and live from an invincible state of mind, you must be ready for the negativity that may come from people you interact with in your life. You also must know how to best protect yourself from energy that can drain you or pull you down. Interestingly, negative commentary, energy, or advice from those closest to you can affect you the most. There are any number of different reasons for this negativity, but it mainly comes down to their own limits of mind or their fear that *your* growth will somehow reflect negatively on who *they* are. As a result, negative or "toxic" people will tell you what can't be accomplished. ("Nobody gets published these days.")

They will try to distract you from your path. ("Come out and party with us tonight. You can always work tomorrow.")

They will give you advice from their more limited, undisciplined, and biased perspective. ("All women just want to use you for your money" or "All men are cheaters.")

They will try to make their beliefs real. ("You're going to lose all your money if you try that.")

They will project their fears on you. ("Making it as a professional [athlete, artist, actor, musician] is a pipe dream. You have to be realistic and get a real job.")

They will try to pull you into confirming their pessimism. ("The world is a mess and is just a horrible place" or "Nobody's happy.")

To be a master creator of your life, you must protect your mind from other people's narrow beliefs. To do this, you must be aware of when this negativity is trying to penetrate your mind and corrupt your optimism. It is OK to listen to constructive criticism from those you respect or embrace the information or words that ring true to you. But never let anyone project a limit on what is possible for you.

You decide what is possible for you.

No matter what your father, mother, siblings, grandparents, relatives, coworkers, or political and religious leaders say, if it's not helpful to your growth and expansion, do not let it affect your mind. Do not get roped into their negative view of the world and their agenda or propaganda. Be ready for any negativity, be grateful your mind doesn't work this way, and move forward with your dreams and desires. *You have to be relentless about maintaining a state of inner peace.* The invincible mindset is about protecting your outlook and state of mind at all costs.

The space between your ears, when connected to your heart, is the most sacred space in the world. When you start to really listen to the stories, advice, and words of those around you, you may be astonished at how negative so many people can be. This is truly poison to the soul. Do not let this affect you, and *stay relentlessly positive. This will serve you best.*

Another trap to be aware of is people who will work to create conflict or drama with you. Some people are simply comfortable with, or even addicted to, conflict and drama. Out of nowhere you may get a text from a family member with a statement or comment that sends your blood pressure soaring, or in a conversation someone may bring up politics or a topic that seems intended to engage you in a negative way. In essence, they are throwing the red cape out, trying to provoke you like how a bullfighter teases a bull. Recognize the cape and do not fall for the trap of engaging in what does not serve you and will only drain your spirit. Conversation is fine, but energy vampires (people who leave you feeling depleted both emotionally and mentally after you've interacted with them) know exactly how to hit weak links and trigger points that work to pull your energy down. Family members can sometimes do this particularly well.

To become more invincible of mind, you must be prepared for this potential energy before you enter a room or conversation. Have a game plan that will prevent you from getting riled up when someone throws out the red cape. Before holidays would be an especially good time to prepare.

- Be ready to face negative comments or be pulled into drama.
- Project an aura of positivity that says, "I AM staying positive and happy."
- If you have not instigated the drama or disagreement, know it is not about you. Do not personalize it, react to it, or give it energy in any way.
- When someone tries to rile you up or bring you down, have compassion and forgive them, for they know not what they do.
- Be grateful for who you are.
- When the triggering energy starts, take a deep breath and ask yourself, "Who do I choose to be now?"
- If there is no way to respond without engaging someone negatively, do not respond at all. Remove yourself from the conversation.

The most powerful thing to remember in these kinds of situations is your ability to reflect on who you choose to be. This will help you regulate your emotions and stick to your choice to stay on the high road. Staying in a higher state of mind and not engaging or contesting makes it much harder for anyone to manipulate you or affect you with their agenda or energy. Stay in this state long enough and you might even positively change them.

> "There are no contests in the art of peace. A true warrior is invincible because he or she contests with nothing."
>
> —Moriche Ueshiba

MASTERING THE TRAP OF UNHEALTHY AND NEGATIVELY PRODUCED NEWS, ENTERTAINMENT, AND SOCIAL MEDIA

As someone looking to be in the greatest mindset each day, you must be vigilant about how you feed your mind. There has been endless talk about how important exercise is to our health. There has been a major focus on the importance of eating healthy and "clean." Sleep training with data trackers on our wrists and the craze of cold plunging have been trends of late for an optimal mindset and improved physical and mental performance. Yet even with all the focus on these methodologies, it is interesting that the mental health crisis has been getting worse every year. It's time to turn the focus to the most important health issue of all: your mind and how to stop feeding it with what has a detrimental effect on your psyche.

Negative news and violence-filled television program-ming and movies are presented to us constantly. They have been a part of the fabric of our culture since television and movies became a part of society. The reality is that fear sells. Now, with a smartphone in everyone's hand and the pro-liferation of social media, our minds are being pummeled with information, videos, and imagery that can have a se-vere impact on our beliefs, perceptions, and state of mind. A heightened understanding of what information is going into your mind is more critical than ever before. We only have to look at the epidemic of debilitating anxiety, depression, fear, addiction, and general unhappiness to see the effect this programming has had on the collective psyche.

When the twenty-four-hour news cycle started over twenty-five years ago, certain cable news channels figured out quickly that the best way to prevent people from changing the channel, and thus keep advertising income and profits high, was to focus on fear-based programming. Basically, the general narrative these networks use is "they're coming to get you, and we'll keep you updated on how you can protect your-self and stop this madness!" The programming they pump out daily tends to be a constant diet of the worst, most horrific stories in the world. Eight billion people are in the global pop-ulation, but certain large news corporations predominantly showcase a skewed view of humanity, along with a narrative that makes viewers feel unsafe, anxious, and angry.

The way news is programmed has a tangible energy as-sociated with it. Sitting and consuming this negative energy every day and night, like so many have done for years, has a corrosive effect on your mind, body, and soul. It shapes your perception, causing you to lose clarity and a sense of confidence in what is true and what isn't. Obviously, it's important to be informed about what's happening in your city, country, and world. The problem arises when you let certain negatively biased entertainment or news channels fill you with bias, false fears, and a negative view of the world. This can cause anxiety and severely affect your mood with family and friends. There's a big, beautiful world out there where wonderful things are happening every day! There are millions of loving, kind people all across the globe.

You can't help the world when you're seeped in the same negative and fear-dominated mindset that is the basis for so much of the suffering. Those who operate from the most balanced and empowered state of mind do not let any news companies' negative narratives manipulate them or corrupt their perspective on life. The best way to get news and stay informed is to find good-quality news sources that have no political agenda. Stay away from news that is programmed to fill you with negative opinions and false rhetoric. Rather than watch the news, I urge you to *read* fact-based, independent reporting from reputable sources. Also, check a few news sources from outside your own country. The more you focus on the evidence-based facts, the more you will protect yourself and your mind from this debilitating and corrosive energy. Remember, optimism and positive energy are the keys to a truly happy life. If these information sources aren't filling your mind with enough of that energy, it's a sign you're being grossly manipulated.

Television programming and movies can also be a source of negative and violent imagery, with violence often being glorified. Constant consumption of this kind of energy can have a very unhealthy effect on your soul. *Dateline, Unsolved Mysteries, Forensic Files, The First 48*, and many other shows on TV and streaming services focus on the most horrible human behaviors. Murders, kidnappings, and other unpleasant situations are showcased from around the world. Consuming this type of programming can generate a lot of subconscious fear and anxiety and can even cause you to be afraid to walk out your front door. This is not to say you should remain ignorant of what is happening in the world. It is about curating what enters your mind and protecting your outlook on society from being inaccurately skewed. Choose your entertainment wisely. Ask yourself, "What do I want to feed my mind today?"

Constant consumption of negative imagery causes your mind to slowly change as you become more fearful, cautious, and unsure about your world. This is the opposite of harnessing the power of life to manifest your greatest power and joy. These programs present situations and ways of thinking that hinder your inner state of peace and hence reduce your outer influence and ability to create good in your life. They are a debilitating trap for your mind.

There are plenty of soul-lifting, energy-boosting TV shows and movies to choose from. Make the commitment to change your mental diet; strengthen your mind, not weaken it; and focus your attention on different and more empowering forms of entertainment.

Social media now dominates a majority of people's attention each day. The average person now spends almost three hours a day scrolling on social media. How could this kind of consumption not have a significant impact on the mind? If you want to stay in the optimal state to tap your infinite potential, it is imperative that you are aware of what imagery is going into your brain every day. Social media is not a good or a bad thing—it is simply the evolutionary result of our efforts to communicate and express who we are as a species. The way to manage this form of mental input is to curate your daily feed so that it improves your mindset. Take the time to cultivate your social media feeds in a way that will help you achieve a more empowered and positive mindset. Do this by seeking out the most educational, joyful, and uplifting content possible. If it doesn't lift your spirit, it's counterproductive to your growth. You have the choice to immediately change this. Use this ability to control your inputs and make sure you monitor how much daily time you give to this medium. Make the commitment to take back control of where you put your attention.

PROTECTING YOUR SACRED STATE OF MIND

The following is a conversation I had with a client whose new success instigated some negative reactions in those close to her. Understanding why such negative reactions occur and being prepared for them is the best way to avoid the trap of engaging with them and falling back into an emotional and unproductive state.

CLIENT: Man, some people always try to rain on a good thing!

ME: Be prepared. As your new positivity and success continue, the naysayers lurk around every corner.

CLIENT: Why is that?

ME: Contrast. Your positivity and success can be difficult for others. Some want only confirmation of their pessimistic point of view. Some don't want to feel worse about themselves. Not that you're making them feel worse, but they just sometimes feel worse in light of your success. It's a survival instinct in a culture of constant comparison.

CLIENT: So I should be careful what I say or who I say it to?

ME: Don't change who you are or your enthusiasm for a minute. Just be prepared for any negative energy or responses. Whether it's friends or family, don't be surprised by any of it.

CLIENT: How do I not react?

ME: You make a commitment to yourself about who you want to be. You decide that no drama, no bad advice, and no small-minded thinking will affect you. The more you're prepared for it, the less susceptible you'll be to it. Stay on high ground.

CLIENT: It can be hard when it's your own father who puts you down or diminishes what you're trying to do.

ME: I understand. However, he doesn't know any different, or he'd offer it. Positivity is often rare and uncharted territory for others. Many of our parents grew up with a lot of negativity and fear. Sometimes it's all they know or experienced. The important thing is for you to protect your optimism and your belief in what is possible. Let your results do the talking for your life. Once you get through people's attempted negativity, you'll likely bring out the best in them!

CLIENT: Boy, that takes some real strength at times. You're right, though. Negativity seems to be everywhere in the world.

ME: Not everywhere. There are also a lot of very positive people in the world. You just have to be prepared for how you want to handle destructive energy when it shows up. You want to keep heading on your path and to your dreams? Be prepared to be absolutely unfazed and undeterred by any sneak attacks on your vibe.

CLIENT: OK. Got it. I'll stay focused. I may not even watch the news anymore—there are so many horrible things happening in the world.

ME: That's not a bad idea. Just remember there are just as many, if not more, positive things happening in the world every day—millions of acts of goodness and kindness you never hear about. It's good to be aware of what's going on in the world so you can take action to help change it. It's about how much what you are focusing on affects you. You just can't let the negative news consume you. Stay aware and compassionate, but also stay in your power. Stay away from the dark side.

THE OPPORTUNITY IN CONFRONTING AND TAKING ON CHALLENGES COURAGEOUSLY

There will be ups and downs and twists and turns on your road to creating a better experience of life. Many days, it can seem like the hurdles and the tests of faith keep coming. The thing to remember is to remain faithful and optimistic. To trust there is always a reason. To never let the circumstances change the power of your belief in what you can accomplish. Challenges give you an incredible opportunity to step up and show life the unrelenting resolve you have about who you are and who you choose to be.

These moments also give you an opportunity to demonstrate that you aren't afraid of anything because you have faith in what will be. Every challenge is seen as a learning opportunity, a growth opportunity, or an opportunity to show that you can and will get through anything. You know you will be stronger and wiser for every experience. This is the invincible mind at its finest.

The often-shared allegory of the white-bearded old captain of the merchant ship from the 1500s comes to mind when talking about a bold way to confront the tests and challenges of life. The captain's ship is in the middle of the ocean, encountering a torrential storm and an extremely rough sea. Waves are crashing across the deck, lightning is flashing, and the crew is nervously bailing the flooding water and making sure the ropes and sails are firm and tight. The captain remains steely eyed at the ship's helm, guiding it as he shouts through the sheets of rain to the men to keep bailing. The waves continue to pound the ship as it rocks back and forth, with the wind whipping through the boat and the thunder cracking louder with each flash of light. The storm seems relentless. Finally, the captain leaves the wheel and goes out to the bow of the boat. Drenched and exhausted, he steadies himself, lifts his arms and fists to the sky, looks up, and yells, "Come on, give me everything ya got!"

At that instant, the storm breaks and the wind and sea settle. Dawn has come.

Within minutes there is a calmness and a deep serenity that can only come after a storm of this magnitude. The ship and crew have made it through the violent thrashing storm and are safe on a peaceful sea again.

This allegory represents the power of the captain's undeterred will. In the middle of the biggest challenge of his life, facing capsizing, drowning, and death, he turned and faced the circumstance with strength and in a way only a seasoned leader and captain could. Life relented to the captain's courageous and powerfully demonstrated faith. He passed the ultimate test, and peace and calm were then restored.

LIVING FROM AN INVINCIBLE STATE OF MIND

How to Walk the Path of Enlightenment, Peace, and Inevitable Success

Thought impregnated with love becomes invincible.

—Charles F. Haanel

Equipped with a new and enriched understanding, you have entered a doorway to an extremely sacred state of being. When you enter this state of awareness, you are in such harmony with life and the perfection of each moment that nothing can disturb your peaceful and graceful state of mind. This is the space of infinite potential and possibilities. In this mindset, you are a master at navigating the universe's ever-shifting winds and tides as you elegantly guide yourself through every ebb and flow of life.

No one can avoid the process of evolving with life. Therefore, the magic of living in the highest state lies in attaining awareness of how to move through each day in harmony with "what is." It is about going into each day with the intention to lift your soul and nurture your creative desires. The soul is fulfilled through purpose, meaning, creativity, passion, understanding, peace, connection, and love. True peace is achieved when you submit to the happenings of life with grace and faith, while still joyfully expressing yourself. To know that life, the universe, truth, consciousness, the Holy Spirit, love, or God (or whatever definition you're comfortable with) is here to continually support you is a comfort that surpasses all knowledge. The power behind this faith is incalculable. Knowing this co-creative relationship is here right now brings the entire universe to your feet.

> "Open your eyes."
> —Opening and closing line
> of Cameron Crowe's film *Vanilla Sky*
> (Paramount Pictures)

YOU ARE THE ULTIMATE OBSERVER

You are the conscious creator of your experience of life from this moment forward. You choose how you will perceive, feel, respond, and therefore affect life. What an astonishing amount of power to decide sits within you!

There are so many in the world who do not know the vast magnitude of this capability, let alone that this ability even exists. Saint Augustine described this almost 1,600 years ago: "Men go abroad to wonder at the heights of mountains, at the huge waves of the sea, at the long courses of the rivers, at the vast compass of the ocean, at the circular motions of the stars, and they pass by themselves without wondering."

Many people remain unaware that a more fulfilling, passionate, and peaceful way of living is one thought and moment away. In so many cases pain and suffering have been normalized, tolerated, and perpetuated.

This can change.

By choosing to bring this awareness into your life, you are honoring yourself and your world beyond measure. You are expanding your energy, your aura, and the impact of your consciousness. You are increasing the brilliance of your light. Nothing you do will carry more meaning than having the will and courage to expand your awareness and your love. Self-awareness is the path to all knowledge and the key to the kingdom. By taking this path, you have truly brought yourself and others in your life a well-deserved gift that benefits the collective consciousness.

"In a land of the blind, the one-eyed man is king."

—Desiderius Erasmus

NEUTRALIZING FEAR

When you are strengthened with new wisdom, one of the only things that can stop you, if you let it, is fear. Fear is the biggest tool the ego uses when faced with change and transformation. It will tell you anything to try to stop you from achieving what you desire and becoming who you know you are destined to be. To neutralize fear and open the door to a timeless way of life, you must summon the power of your will. Your will for change, combined with the awareness that your negative, self-limiting thoughts are *valueless lies*, is what will help you overcome fear. Fear is insidious because it works by projecting the worst possible outcomes as your destined truth.

"He who fears he shall suffer, already suffers what he fears."

—Michel de Montaigne

The real truth is that there is an infinite spectrum of possibilities that includes the optimal results you can imagine for yourself.

By interviewing for the job you want, you might get the

job and have a rewarding career for a lifetime. By asking the person you are interested in out on a date, you might actually convince them to say yes, which could lead to a lifetime of love and companionship. By playing, practicing, or trying out for the team, you might perform at the highest level, make the team, and gain a new level of confidence for the rest of your life. By making the appointment and going to the doctor, you might get the test results that finally give you complete peace of mind. By asking your customer or prospect for an order, you might get the biggest order in your company's history and forever be unafraid to think from a bigger perspective.

Here is why fear is counterproductive to creating the life you dream of: the instigating thought of any fear is your belief that the negative thought you are having is true. If this was not the case, the thought and fear wouldn't have any energetic effect on you. In step three, you learned that you consciously and subconsciously shape your reality toward what you believe is true. Life, in turn, works to validate your beliefs whether they are positive or negative. Carrying fear in your mind does not help you achieve what you desire. Fear works to destroy what you desire.

This is not to say that fear does not have a purpose. It certainly does. It helps you stay away from danger and risks to your existence. But the fear that stops you from becoming who you want to be, and experiencing what you desire to do, is valueless. Fear is completely counterproductive to the intent to live life fully and be in the invincible state of existence.

Faith, on the other hand, works to create your desires. Consider this observation from the legendary pitcher Sandy Koufax: "I became a good pitcher when I stopped trying to make them miss the ball and started trying to make them hit it." Embedded in this statement is the power of faith over fear. Koufax's focus on trying to make batters miss stemmed from his fear that they would hit the ball. When he dropped his fear of the batter making contact and embraced faith in his pitches and a positive outlook, he became a great pitcher.

Do not confuse faith with certainty. *Faith does not mean certainty in the outcome—it means trust in any outcome, whatever it may be.* It means you have a sense of peace about your preparation and process to achieve any result. This allows you to stay peaceful and mindful about the process. Having faith is not an expectation of your desired result but a feeling of trust that you are doing all you can for your desired intent to become real. Nothing is certain in life. That is the beauty of life and the real test of faith.

On the other side of fear is faith.

One of the greatest examples I've ever seen of mastery over fear is the story and accomplishments of rock climber Alex Honnold. The documentary on his incredible feat, *Free Solo*, won the Academy Award for Best Documentary Feature Film in 2019. In the film, directors Jimmy Chin and Elizabeth Chai Vasarhelyi document Alex's quest to climb the famous three-thousand-foot wall named El Capitan in Yosemite National

Park. Oh, and did I mention that he did this nearly four-hour vertical climb without a single safety rope? He had nothing to save him from falling. A missed step, a lapse in mental focus, or a bad fingernail hold and it was all over.

What Alex Honnold accomplished is not only one of the greatest athletic feats in history but one of the greatest examples of what the human mind can achieve. For almost four hours, dangling on the side of a mountain, Alex executed a supreme faith in who he was and how well he had prepared to accomplish his athletic goal. In Alex's case, the cost of not executing one single move would lead to his death. He inspired millions by sharing what is possible when you harness the power of the mind, possibility, focus, preparation, planning, patience, determination, will, and courage. Basically, he demonstrated the invincible state of mind and the power of absolute faith. In doing so, he showed so many people what is possible and what they can accomplish in their own lives by learning to stay in the very focused, mindful, and precise moment-by-moment process at hand. While very few people on the earth will ever "free solo" the vertical side of a three-thousand-foot mountain, everyone deals with fear in some aspect of their lives. The process of mastering it is the same.

When it comes to overcoming fear and accomplishing what you desire, staying in the moment is critical because it doesn't leave any room for you to think. Thinking can be dangerous because it can lead to the projection of a certain outcome. Projection can lead to doubt. Doubt is destructive and opens the door to fear and a racing mind that steals precious time and focus. In Alex Honnold's case, doubt would have meant death. He showed the power of faith and focus and demonstrated that faith is built through belief, preparation, planning, and practice down to every minute detail. This is what kept him in the process of executing the intricate handholds and body positions of elite-level climbing. He was focused only on each calculated small move forward. To allow his mind to wander from his next fingerhold or toe crimp would distract him. By laser focusing his mind only on his next move and not getting ahead of himself, he eventually achieved what was believed to be the impossible.

Every great athlete, entertainer, or businessperson who became a master at their craft has developed a similar mindset; they learned to stay laser focused on the process at hand in a way that keeps moving them closer and closer to their dreams.

> "Success usually comes to those who are too
> busy to be looking for it."
> —Henry David Thoreau

THE POWER OF INTENDING INSTEAD OF EXPECTING

One of the most useful distinctions I teach the top-level athletes I coach is the difference between *intending* and *expecting*. In 2015 I was working with one of the top pitchers in Major League Baseball. In one stretch of the season, he was having trouble executing outs with batters in the seventh, eighth, and ninth hitting positions in the batting order. He asked, "Why have I been struggling with the weaker hitters in the lineup?" My response was, "That answer is found in your question." He was making an assumption that was leading him to an expectation. This expectation was taking him out of his most focused state of mind. The assumption was that the seventh, eighth, and ninth hitters were "weak" hitters. I asked him, "Do you remember what kind of talent it takes for a player to get himself into a Major League lineup?" He immediately knew where I was going with this question. The hitters he was facing in these positions were still some of the best hitters in the world. He had to acknowledge this because nothing can be taken for granted when you want to operate at the highest level. By assuming these players were easier outs, his mind embraced the expectation that he *should get them out*, rather than staying respectful, mindful, and in the locked-in mindset of *intending to get them out*. This state produces the highest probability of selecting the best pitches to throw these players in order to win the matchup. We see it all the time in sports when players on a powerful team meet a big underdog and assume or expect they are going to win. The better team takes the underdog too lightly, thus setting them up to be thrown off-balance if things don't go their way. Hence, the team becomes ripe for the upset.

The lesson is to be extremely mindful when either competing in sports or creating anything in your life. The most powerful place of mind to stay in is the process of intention.

This focus keeps your mind, body, and soul working in harmony to achieve your intention. Expectation, however, puts your mind on the future and takes you slightly out of the process. "Slightly" is all it takes to lose the edge.

As you learned in step one, one of life's main intentions is to meet ignorance with life-sustaining awareness. The meaning of *life-sustaining* is based on how you intend to create and survive. Life must reveal all limiting or destructive beliefs that could prevent you from manifesting your exact intention. Expecting, and putting a conclusive limit on, the truth of infinite possibilities destines you to learn that anything is possible. In other words, you're destined to what you didn't expect! Intending keeps you just humble enough to stay focused, attentive, and locked into your creative process.

A present without humility leads to a future with suffering.

If you want to be the best pitcher in the world, life will have to make you aware of how to do it. If you assume certain hitters are weak, the bottom three hitters will have success over you until you learn to treat them with enough respect, stay completely focused, and properly execute during the matchup. Assume or expect nothing, and instead, *intend to fearlessly pitch your best.*

If you want to have the most fulfilling relationship possible, take nothing for granted. Stay in the space of intending that experience with your significant other by participating in the daily fun, love, and care that nurtures this type of relationship. *Intend to have the most loving connection possible.*

If you want to be the best employee, don't expect your boss to promote you or give you a raise just because you feel that you're irreplaceable. Instead, intend to be the best employee *by consistently working harder and smarter,* and trust that the rest will take care of itself.

REALIZING YOUR IMMORTALITY

What if you knew your existence was never in doubt? The effect on how you'd go through life would be astonishing. The power of your presence would amplify. No longer hyperfocused on yourself in each moment, you would be free to use your full attention to see how your presence could help those around you. Because of this new presence, your ability to anticipate or intuit what's going to happen would skyrocket. You'd unlock the mind of a master-level chess player. Next-level mindfulness would then take on an entirely new meaning. With the awareness of the late, great athlete Muhammad Ali, you would see almost every one of life's swings and punches coming before they even happened. You would dance and float through life, creating as you intend. You would be open to all possibilities. A liberated mind is an invincible soul that shines brightly.

Freedom from the idea of death is the freedom to live fearlessly.

By seeing your eternal nature, you diminish the influence of fear in your life. When you peel all the layers of the onion back, you see that all your fears are linked to the fear of not existing. That is why when you can't validate who you believe that you are, your ego goes into red alert mode. Two things are critical to remember here. One, since you are the eternal observer of life, your existence is never in doubt. You must go on. The form your consciousness will take may change, but you will continue to be. Have you ever known yourself to not exist? And two, the more you accept difficult change, the easier you will adjust and navigate your way through these times with less suffering and more faith and grace.

Seeing death as a doorway to another yet-to-be-known experience, rather than an end, is ironically one of the keys to a limitless experience here and now. When you contemplate the truth of an infinite universe and you combine it with the reality that energy is neither created nor destroyed, you can begin to see the truth of your own spiritual immortality. Your consciousness is beyond the boundaries of beginning and end. You are an infinite essence revealed in a finite expression, destined to experience the truth of all forms. You are continually prodded and nudged into an inspired sense of movement, encouraged to evolve by the winds of an endlessly changing and expanding universe. Your life is a never-ending experience of creative expression, expansion, evolvement, and transformation where anything is possible.

The question to ask yourself in terms of faith in your continual existence, whatever form this may take, is, "How can

I not have faith?" To make it to this moment in your life, you have survived every one of your fearful "How am I going to get through this?" experiences. The universe has never abandoned you and it never will. You are linked together in an eternal co-creative cosmic relationship. Physical death is just another doorway of transformation to a new experience. Like the caterpillar that enters the portal of the cocoon and comes out the other side transformed into a beautiful butterfly, your life force will go on and evolve.

In the meantime, your existence itself demonstrates there is a profound reason for it or you wouldn't be here now. Stay faithful. You matter. You have more life to live, lessons to learn, love to give and receive, and other lives to touch. Everything you need is in the here and now. There is so much opportunity to use the grace of mental and physical existence that has been gifted to you to find the true "heaven on earth." Whenever the divine universe determines it's your "time" to transcend to a new experience is when it's your time. Physical death is not an end but rather a doorway to another new adventure.

TRUSTING THAT THERE IS TIME

With an open mind and belief in your infinite self, you perceive time less as a stressor and a limited commodity. Less panicked, hurried, fearful, and needful, you settle into the moment and see more of the bigger picture. *Relax and take a big, freeing breath. You're exactly where you're supposed to be now; there is no other place in space or time. Everything is still in front of you!*

Not worrying about time doesn't make you more wasteful of it; this actually enriches your experience so that you get more quality out of each moment. Why? Because the peace this understanding gives you allows you to enjoy more of what's happening around you. Music sounds better, laughter comes easier, food tastes richer, and flowers smell sweeter. Sunrises and sunsets seem more beautiful than ever before. Living more timelessly increases your sense of calm and allows you to be fully present. Presence enhances your memory and increases the manifestation power of your intentions.

> "Don't let the fear of the time it will take to
> accomplish something stand in the way of
> your doing it. The time will pass anyway."
> —Earl Nightingale

NEEDING NOTHING

I believe the Buddha's words may have been misinterpreted over 2,500 years ago when he said, "Desire is the root of all suffering." Desire is not the root of suffering. For human beings, it is natural and healthy to have desires. Desires can be exciting. Desire is a very natural part of life's creative process. *The root of all suffering, it turns out, is not desire but need.*

When you have a need such "as I need that job," or "I

need that relationship," or "I need this win," you are acting from a state of lack and fear. You may feel somehow incomplete or fear being unable to survive without what you feel you "need." This does not mean you can't have wants, dreams, and desires, but when you move to a fear-based feeling of need, you are immediately in a state of misunderstanding and are thus suffering. This is the lie. As an incarnation from a divine universe, you are perfectly complete just as you are.

The proper state of mind and the one that will keep you most creatively empowered is "I don't need this job, but I would like to have this job." If you go into a job interview with this outlook, you will have a sense of calmness and confidence, which you won't have if you go into the interview in a state of need. Going into a relationship with a sense of need is never a good thing. Need will make you jealous, controlling, and, well, needy. Confidence (not cockiness) is what is sexy and attractive. Desiring the relationship, however, is perfectly fine. Needing to win or perform in sports creates stress and diminishes your talent and performance. *Desiring* or *intending* to do well, and even the sacred place of knowing you're going to do well, keeps you in the best space to let your true talent shine unobstructed.

> "A Zen master observing students at archery practice notices one of them who is consistently missing the mark and says, 'He thinks more of winning than of shooting and the need to win drains him of power.'"
>
> —Chaung Tzu

Because need stems from fear, you are already in a weak state of energy and working against yourself. In this state of mind, your poisoning destructive belief is "I can't" or "I won't." *Don't need—instead intend with trust and faith that when the conditions are finally right, what you want will become a reality.* This way of thinking puts you in the most powerful state of energy possible. The needle of probability then moves in favor of your desires materializing. The empowered mind has the ability to let go of the outcome enough to rest in the place of knowing that regardless of what happens, everything will be all right. Thus, you enter a state of true grace with a clear mind and soul that enable you to create effortlessly.

> "The bird of paradise lands only on the hand
> that does not grasp."
>
> —Zen proverb

FEARLESS WILL AND RELENTLESS PERSISTENCE

The will to act on your dreams and at the same time be open to continually learn is what will put you in flow. You must consistently demonstrate who you believe you are and what you believe is possible through action and the fortitude to never give up. Knowing you cannot fail but can only learn is very liberating to the mind and adds energy and enthusiasm to your actions. This resolve is your creative strength.

"Strength does not come from physical ca-
pacity. It comes from an indomitable will."
　　　　　　　　　　—Mahatma Gandhi

When you are empowered with the understanding of
unlimited self-worth and the energy of resolute action, it is
only a matter of time before you put all the necessary conditions together. It's important that you are able to envision
yourself attaining what you desire without hesitation. This
is when fear is overcome and you start to take action toward
new results that you may have never thought possible before.

Belief is extremely powerful, but its power can only be
unleashed by a mind that removes limitation and increases
self-worth. Belief is also known as hope, and it has been
scientifically demonstrated that hope increases resolve and
determination. Human beings throughout history have
been known to do extraordinary things and achieve mind-
boggling results using the power of belief. You are capable
and worthy of so much more!

"Nothing in the world can take the place of
persistence. Talent will not; nothing is more
common than unsuccessful men with talent.
Genius will not; unrewarded genius is almost
a proverb. Education will not; the world is
full of educated derelicts. Persistence and determination alone are omnipotent."
　　　　　　　　　　—Calvin Coolidge

THE CHAMPION MINDSET

Below is a collection of quotes from some of the most accomplished athletes in the world. These individuals have manifested results from a mindset of infinite possibility and have in turn inspired millions of people through their efforts. What is so interesting about these particular quotes is that every single one of them is relatable to anything you are trying to accomplish in your life. They are treasured pieces of wisdom.

"I don't think limits."

—Usain Bolt,
eight-time Olympic gold medalist sprinter
and world record holder

"I'm a very positive thinker and I always see the good in life."

—Roger Federer,
former world number one tennis player
and winner of twenty Grand Slam
championship titles

"Success for me is knowing that I've given absolutely everything that I can."

—Ashleigh Barty,
former world number one tennis player and
three-time Grand Slam singles champion

"You can't be afraid to fail. It's the only way to succeed."

—LeBron James,
four-time world champion basketball player
and all-time leading scorer in the NBA

"Make sure your worst enemy doesn't live between your own two ears."

—Laird Hamilton, world-renowned
big-wave surfer, inventor, and innovator

"Stay healthy, have fun, and embrace all the moments because anything can happen."

—Simone Biles,
the greatest gymnast of all time
and the most decorated in US history

"Of all the hazards, fear is the worst."

—Sam Snead,
former PGA Tour professional,
tied for the most professional victories
in PGA Tour golf history

"I think your mind really controls everything."

—Michael Phelps,
world champion swimmer and the
most decorated Olympic athlete in history,
with twenty-three gold medals

"Everybody believes in something. Most of all we should believe in ourselves."

—Novak Djokovic,
ranked eight times as the world's
number one tennis player,
holder of a record twenty-four
Grand Slam championship titles, and
Olympic gold medal winner

"I may win, and I may lose, but I will never be defeated."

—Emmitt Smith,
all-time leading rusher in NFL history
and three-time Super Bowl champion

"I think self-awareness is the most important thing to becoming a champion."

—Billie Jean King,
one of the greatest tennis players of all time
and holder of thirty-nine Grand Slam titles

"You can knock me down, but I will get up twice as strong."

—Lewis Hamilton,
Formula One driver with seven
World Drivers' Championship titles
and multiple world records

"Never say never, because limits, like fears, are often an illusion."

> —Michael Jordan,
> six-time NBA champion and
> the greatest basketball player of all time

"I've learned to become my own biggest cheerleader, always feeding myself positive thoughts, visualizing myself winning, and most importantly focusing on each individual point."

> —Ibtihaj Muhammad,
> world champion Olympic fencer

"Concentration and mental toughness are the margins of victory."

> —Bill Russell, winner of eleven
> NBA championships and one of the greatest
> basketball players of all time

"Technique and ability alone do not get you to the top; it is the willpower that is the most important. This willpower you cannot buy with money or be given by others . . . it rises from your heart."

> —Junko Tabei, first woman to reach
> the summit of Mount Everest

"If you want to perform at the highest level, you have to prepare at the highest level mentally."

—Tom Brady,
seven-time Super Bowl champion
and greatest NFL quarterback of all time

"I really think a champion is defined not by their wins but by how they can recover when they fall."

—Serena Williams,
winner of a record twenty-three
Grand Slam singles championship titles and
one of the greatest tennis players of all time

"Impossible is nothing."

—Muhammed Ali,
the greatest boxer of all time

"Giving up is never in the equation."

—Tiger Woods,
winner of fifteen major championships
and one of the greatest golfers of all time

One of the most interesting comments I've ever heard about an athlete came from a sportswriter who was talking about Tiger Woods. He said that Tiger Woods's opponents have never been people. *His main opponent has always been history*. Tiger's top priority was not as much about defeating his opponents as it was looking at the much bigger picture of conquering history by becoming the greatest player who ever lived. This aspiration and the energy of this intention are a major part of what took him to a level of will, determination, and play that superseded that of any other competitor he faced for years. It is this massive goal, and the consistent actions that followed it, that carried him to his greatness and his legendary status as an athlete. The moral of the story is that small plans will yield small results. If you really want to achieve something, you cannot be afraid to dream it as big as you possibly can.

MASTER-LEVEL MINDSET

An invincible mind is a very efficient mind because it is focused on fully accepting where you are, finding out what needs to be done next, and working intently on gathering the information regarding how you do it. The invincible mind does not resist any of life's challenges; it meets them with the same patience and faith that you feel when life is going smoothly.

When you have a mindset of infinite potential, you understand that the human experience is one of many twists and turns. Your mind has to be ready for them in terms of strategy and response. Having this state of mind is like being a top Formula One race car driver. Elite-level drivers are the very best at being able to anticipate the rough spots and twists and turns on the road ahead. They have practiced, visualized, and prepared for it all. They are able to see these challenges as early as possible, and they know how to turn into them and steer through them with world-class efficiency so they don't lose control or crash. They come out of the twists and turns rapidly and with little lost time or damage, and they get up to top speed again in an instant. It is the same when you are striving to live in the most powerful state of mind.

To have an invincible state of mind, you must be highly prepared, aware, and fearless. To be fearless, you must be faithful. You can't take the risk out of life. At some point you must be vulnerable and demonstrate faith. This is a faith in life and in something greater than yourself that sustains your soul as it pulls you through evolution and time. Building this kind of connection with life will serve you in incalculable ways in the future. Understanding this relationship now is so much better than waiting until you are faced with one of life's bigger challenges, which can throw you off-balance and put you in a state of emotional desperation.

The main questions it all comes down to right now are:

- Do you want to be truly happy right now?
- Do you want to feel fulfilled and at peace even as you work to achieve more?
- Do you want the vision and mindset that allow you to excel at achieving any desire?

- Do you want to be the master of your own mind and be impervious to negativity and the suffering it causes?

If the answer is yes to any of these questions, there is only one thing left to do:

Prove it.

Demonstrate that you see your infinite potential by how inspired you feel each morning and by dreaming big.

Show how much you understand yourself by exhibiting honesty, love, and compassion to yourself every day.

Express gratitude by believing you are worthy of feeling blessed every day.

Validate your worth by taking action toward achieving what you want and becoming who you want to be.

Exhibit the love you feel toward life for getting you here by giving back to your world each day and treating others with kindness and compassion.

Don't let what hasn't happened yet in your life affect what could happen.

Statistics and percentages are *meaningless to a person who believes in who they are in this moment.* This is why people who make decisions and coach solely on analytics in sports are working against themselves. In this infinite moment you can throw out what *has* happened. Probabilities are being formed by the belief of the individual or team in every moment of action.

There is a great moment in the movie *Star Wars: The Empire Strikes Back* when Han Solo is trying to get away from Darth Vader. He flies his ship into an asteroid field to evade him, and the robot C-3PO says, "Sir, the possibility of successfully navigating an asteroid field is approximately 3,720 to 1!" Han Solo replies, "Never tell me the odds."

It doesn't matter what you are facing right now. What matters is how much belief you have in what you can accomplish and how you demonstrate this belief in every moment. The true champion of life stays in the field of all possibilities because in each moment anything is possible!

YOU MAKE YOUR OWN ODDS

Regardless of anything that's happened in the past, everything can change tomorrow. You're never too old and it's never too late to be who you want to be. It's about the consistency of your beliefs in action. Freedom of mind is found in fearlessly walking into whatever is in front of you with the knowledge that it's all going to be OK. It always has been, and it always will be.

As you get older, you can get conservative, protective, and defensive in nature. In order to stay young of heart and vibrant of mind, you must keep your mind open to hope, inspiration, and what is possible every day. This optimistic, open attitude creates the energy that keeps you learning, growing, and living to the fullest. When working to make your dreams a reality, you must encourage yourself to take a step toward your goal every day not only because this is a key to creating what you want, but because you are generating the energy of purpose. That is the real energy behind what's working to create your future. The real key to staying young at heart is maintaining the creative inspiration and movement that comes from optimism and never losing sight of the infinite potential before you.

> "Young people do not know enough to be
> prudent and therefore attempt the impossible
> and achieve it generation after generation."
> —Pearl S. Buck

DECLARING YOUR PERSONAL CREED

Any major vision you have for what you want to accomplish or experience in your life accelerates when you develop a personal creed. A personal creed is a list of guiding principles or beliefs. Developing a creed is like plugging in a destination on your GPS. It sets you on the path to becoming who you desire to be. *It is your daily reminder, map, and compass based on the life you want for yourself.* It helps you find your true north in terms of the energy and attitude you want to carry through life.

Below is a checklist of things to keep in mind for writing your creed:

- Your creed should consist of a minimum of seven core statements of who you are, who you desire to be, or what you desire to accomplish every day.
- Write them as "I AM," "I AM becoming . . . ," or "I AM dedicated to . . ." statements.
- The list should reflect what defines you, your values as a person, and your daily actions.
- When reading your creed, you should feel in exact alignment with it, and the list should give you an inspirational boost in your mind and soul.

Take the time to write your personal creed right now.

TAKE INSPIRED ACTION

Once you have written your creed, the next step is to begin to act on your intentions. You should immediately investigate any hesitation so you can discover the source of your resistance. If there is *any* resistance, you will find a limiting belief lurking somewhere in your consciousness. Identify it as quickly as possible and dissolve it by presenting yourself with a stronger self-defining statement that counters any limit and aligns with your intention.

> "You don't know how paralyzing it is, that stare from a blank canvas that says to the painter, 'You can't do anything.' The canvas has an idiotic stare and mesmerizes some painters so that they turn into idiots themselves. Many painters are afraid of the blank canvas, but the blank canvas is afraid of the truly passionate painter who dares and has once broken the spell of 'you can't.'"
>
> —Vincent van Gogh

The moment of action or inaction on your newly stated self-declarations is your moment of truth. It reveals the level of your intent, belief, desire, will, and faith. Taking action should feel seamless, exciting, and fulfilling. Any other feeling reveals that you are not ready to move forward yet. Inaction indicates that fears are still preventing you from moving forward. You cannot outrun your truth. If fears are part of your current beliefs, these fears will cast a dark shadow over your life until you decide to acknowledge them, dissolve them, and walk into the light of possibility.

"Every shadow, no matter how deep, is threatened by the morning light."
—Line from Darren Aronofsky's film
The Fountain (Warner Bros.)

CHOOSING AN EMPOWERING PERSPECTIVE

What if instead of letting the lie of fear rule any of your creative thoughts, you wake up in the morning and your first words become, "What good is going to happen to me today?" This is a powerful shift of perspective. Actually, embracing this one simple idea with complete authenticity and unbridled optimism can completely change your life. *Own your narrative, and in turn, own the space around you.* If you don't own the space energetically and authentically regarding what you intend to create and who you are, rest assured someone else's dominant energy will. The narrative demonstrated by your state of mind and actions has to be stronger than any of your fears. This state of mind has to be stronger than anyone else's negativity or anyone else's agenda. When you go out into your day, walk into a room or a business meeting, compete in an event, ask someone out, or work your craft, know who you are and what you bring to the space. Then fully own it energetically and mentally with every single fiber of your being.

Whenever you feel inspired by the thought of some amazing possibility for your future, ask yourself this simple and very profound question:

Why not me?

If any objections arise in your mind in response to this question, acknowledge them and then replace them with the truth.

You are worthy.

You are deserving.

You are capable.

Any objections to these are lies. Choose to no longer listen to the lies.

So many people are mentally defeated by fear, worry, and limitation because they don't know their true worth. So many doubt their worth to the point that their dreams remain just that, a dream.

You now know your worth and the creative power that you have been endowed with. You can start your life completely anew in this very moment. Start it with this extremely powerful mantra: I *can* and I *will* because I AM.

Whatever it is, whatever your heart truly desires, repeat this statement and then act.

I can and I will because I AM.

The fear of failure or imperfection has stifled the best-laid plans of millions of people throughout history. Choose to be free of limitation and negative projection. Choose to see only the beauty of what can be in this very moment. Choose to be mentally invincible.

THE EIGHT STATES OF CONSCIOUS CREATION

Attaining the invincible mind is a process of implementing eight states of consciousness into your daily life. Each state on the following list has an important verifying question that goes along with it. Use this checklist as a guide to reveal what to focus on next in the process of building an invincible mind.

1. **The state of readiness.** Readiness opens your mind to receive the enlightenment necessary to break any undesired patterns in your life and accelerate the path to self-mastery. Readiness starts the process of drawing new insights into your mind.

    Are you truly ready for the change you desire?

2. **The state of self-awareness.** Self-awareness ends resistance to any of your past choices and brings clarity and understanding to every previous moment of your life.

    Are you aware of how you have subconsciously and consciously created and are creating your life?

3. **The state of self-realization.** Self-realization reveals your unlimited worth. This brings forth the self-respect and self-love that completely fill your soul and fuel your will to create.

    Are you aware of your infinite worth?

4. **The state of infinite potential.** Embracing infinite possibility allows you to see that there are no limits on you.

   Are you aware of the infinite potential in every moment?

5. **The state of intention ("I AM").** Intention is the magic wand of creation. Understanding this power within you is key to being a master creator of your life.

   Are you aware of the power of "I AM" within you?

6. **The state of humility.** Humility is the doorway to wisdom, and wisdom keeps you in the state of awareness and grace.

   Are you aware there is always more to know and learn?

7. **The state of persistence.** Persistence is a requirement of creation. The will to consistently demonstrate the belief in who you are in the pursuit of your desires is paramount to the invincible mindset.

   Are you willing to persevere in your efforts no matter what challenge is presented to you?

8. **The state of faith.** Faith is the crowning demonstration of the invincible mind and the magic elixir of the process of creation. Faith reveals your true knowledge.

Do you completely trust the process of life, no matter the circumstance or outcome?

How did you do on those answers? If you hesitated or couldn't answer with an emphatic yes, dive into the question to try to find out why you answered this way. Figuring this out and finding the truth are critical to this new mindset. Take a moment now to look back at your answers to the reflection questions from the first four steps in part one of the book. How have your responses evolved? How have your awareness and perspective changed?

Each of the eight states *embraced* represents an exponential shift in your consciousness. All of these states achieved together are the attainment of the invincible mind. This energy opens the door to all of life's possibilities and shifts the needle of probability closer to everything you desire to experience. *All that is left is your devoted persistence and patience.*

Remember, there are no guarantees in life. Understanding this is true faith. Life will vet each person for their understandings. Those who demonstrate humility, acceptance, and patience—the tenets of faith—will be shown favor. These are the traits of true self-mastery.

There is a well-known Zen story of a student who went to a teacher and declared that he wanted to attain enlightenment, saying he was devoted and ready. He asked, "How long would it take?" The teacher replied, "Ten years." Impatient and not satisfied with the answer, the student said, "But

I want to achieve enlightenment faster than that. I will work very hard. I will meditate for ten or more hours a day if necessary. How long would it then take?" The teacher replied, "Twenty years."

This story conveys the wisdom of knowing what it takes to get out of your own way. Need, impatience, lack of contemplation and reflection, and lack of acceptance and faith all lead to more suffering and time.

WHAT TO DO NOW

This exact moment is always the most opportune moment to take complete control over your experience of reality. Life is meant to be lived. Go live your truth. Reach for your dreams. Create the amazing reality you are worthy of living. Dive into the power of infinite potential.

CLIENT: So what you are saying is that anything is possible with the understanding of true mindfulness?

ME: Yes, absolutely! We see it every day in the displays of endless creativity and ingenuity around the globe. We have been incredible at creating new possibilities in the material world. I'd say it's long past time for us to focus on advancing what is mentally and spiritually possible as well. It's time to learn how to raise our consciousness and understanding of the power of goodness and love that is in each one of us. The positive change that can emerge from this knowledge is beyond measurable. The world seems to be craving it.

CLIENT: It feels so overwhelming to know this power is in each of us.

ME: While it can feel overwhelming at times, *humbling* may be a better word. Remember, there is no obligation or responsibility to do anything with this knowledge. Use this insight and wisdom in your own time and at your own pace. Create however you'd like, big or small.

CLIENT: That feels better. I just want to make sure I do a good job honoring what I've learned.

ME: You cannot fail. There is no judgment. To feel most in harmony with life, just follow your heart and spread kindness and joy. That intent will never lead you astray. Keep the faith that life knows best about what opportunities to present. It's all about the endless journey of awareness. A journey with no destination. There is always more to know and understand. Just take it one day and one moment at a time.

CLIENT: Where do I start? What do I do?

ME: You've already started! You're doing it right here, right now, by bringing this insight into your awareness. Now you go back into your life with this newfound understanding and self-appreciation. Set your intention, ask your questions in earnest, and then follow the path, wherever your expanded heart leads you. This new perspective on yourself and life will produce all sorts of wonderful new outcomes on your road ahead.

KNOWING TRUE GRACE

You are now ready to continue your walk with a renewed spirit of mind and a heart full of self-compassion, love, and respect. The tests may come, but you are more prepared to deal with them than ever before. Make the commitment to shine your light and love and not allow the negativity of the world to throw you off-balance under any circumstance. For it has been said in different ways and forms for centuries that light can never be overcome by darkness, but darkness is always overcome by the light.

The following are some wise quotes from wonderful, grace-filled human beings who have significantly influenced the greater consciousness of the world.

> "You cannot get through a single day without
> having an impact on the world around you."
> —Jane Goodall

> "Faith in oneself is the best and safest course."
> —Michelangelo

> "I lead from the heart, not the head."
> —Diana, Princess of Wales

> "May your choices reflect your hopes, not
> your fears."
> —Nelson Mandela

"Whoever is happy will make others happy. He who has courage and faith will never perish in misery!"

—Anne Frank

"Not all of us can do great things. But we can do small things with great love."

—Mother Teresa

"Our own self-realization is the greatest service we can render the world."

—Ramana Maharshi

"Radiate boundless love towards the entire world."

—The Buddha

The power in you is omnipotent. With this awareness, you are ready to create your life experience at will. To gather momentum, you may have to wait at times for the wind to blow and the tide to shift, but by having your sail ready, you'll be prepared for every circumstance and every opportunity to gain speed when the conditions favor you. Divine timing will have its say, but you can chart the course and steer your life by demonstrating who you choose to be every day and by trusting life at every turn.

Along your journey, remember to accept and respect the reality of change and you'll be ready for it before it arrives.

The grace of this knowledge, when applied, will bring you untold riches of experience and the realization of many of your deepest dreams. It will bring you to a place of mind that is beyond description. A place where you see all of life as one interconnected dance. A place where all is one and one is all. Share this wealth of knowledge with your world. Lift others up and stay positive and optimistic no matter how difficult the world can seem at times. Trust that there is a divine order within life's seeming chaos. Continue to contribute your love and wisdom everywhere you can. It truly matters.

> "Don't spend your precious time asking why the world isn't a better place; it will only be time wasted. The question to ask is: How can I make the world better? To that there is an answer."
>
> —Leo Buscaglia

The glittering gold of truth, answers, and peace of mind, the true stairway to heaven, is always as close to you as the whispering wind. With a mindset of infinite potential, "success," however you define this, is inevitably yours. As a result of this new mindset, may your life overflow with love, and may that love and the strength, empathy, and gentleness of your expanded awareness positively affect your world and every single life you touch. May you feel the blessing and joy of an invincible mind and indomitable spirit all the days of your life!

Invincible

No one ever told me
What life was here to show me.
A maze where I felt blind,
A puzzle that wasn't defined.

The search was never out there,
The path always right here.
A power I've already had.
Spirituality is not a fad.

So proud I kept persisting.
No truth is worth resisting.
Life has just been priming.
Patient with divine timing.

This story is finally my making.
I'm blessed so much I'm shaking.
Creation now flows freely,
Propelled by love so deeply.

I now know who I AM.
Nothing can take away my plans.
Graced with the peace of infinite knowing.
My next moment will be my showing.

Acknowledgments

There are so many people whom I have had the honor of working with and teaching this wisdom to that have contributed in one way or another to this book. To all the athletes and individuals I have had or have the grace of helping, guiding, and coaching, I am grateful for all of you.

I'd like to thank my literary agent Stephany Evans for her incredible guidance and wisdom; Stephanie Gunning for her trusted professional editorial eye; Glenn Yeffeth for his faith in my work; Victoria Carmody for her wonderful editorial help and care; and all the wonderful people at BenBella Books for their support, professionalism, enthusiasm, and deep conviction in this work.

To my wife, life-partner, and soulmate, Beth, your unwavering faith, support, and love is such an immeasurable part of this book coming into being. My gratitude and love for you are impossible to put into words. To my two greatest gifts, Sydney and Jeffrey, you inspire and make me proud to be your father every single day. To my father, Edwin Falco, thank you for showing me what it is to keep a beautiful sense of humor about life throughout all of the ups and downs. And of course, to my mother, Maureen Buley, who is a part of everything I AM and who I know is continually guiding me from above.

And lastly, to you, the reader of these words. Thank you for opening to this material and integrating it as a part of your life's path. May this book and its message contribute to your life being lived from the highest state of peace, love, and joy every single day.

About the Author

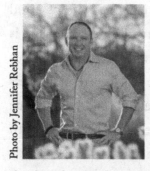

Photo by Jennifer Rebhan

Howard Falco is a mental strength coach and modern-day spiritual teacher. He is also an author and a speaker on the nature of mindfulness, reality, and the power of the mind. Howard has worked to successfully empower the minds of hundreds of college and professional athletes, including those in Major League Baseball, the NFL, the NBA, and the PGA and LPGA Tours. He has also worked with CEOs, corporate executives, and everyday individuals looking for a new way of overcoming life's challenges and achieving new results. His first book was *I AM: The Power of Discovering Who You Really Are* (Tarcher/Penguin, 2010). His second book was *Time in a Bottle: Mastering the Experience of Life* (Tarcher/Penguin, 2014).

In 2002, at age thirty-five, Howard experienced a sudden and massive expansion of mind that left him with a clear understanding of the creative power of life and the origins of all human joy and suffering. During his enlightenment, the reason behind all human creation, action, and inaction was revealed to him. Stunned and inspired by this powerful knowledge, Howard set out to honor this insight by sharing what he learned and teaching others how to attain the most optimal state of mind for personal creation.

Through his work, Howard guides individuals to new, liberating insights and self-awareness that help them remove fear, break through limits, and achieve new results. The intention is to offer a more powerfully creative state of mind that leads to a new desired personal reality. His message is that regardless of the current circumstance we find ourselves in, we all have the same access to the wisdom that answers our deepest questions, changes our reality, and brings true inner peace. We only have to realize that each of us is both capable and worthy of experiencing this.

Howard grew up in Chicago, graduated from Arizona State University, and lives in Arizona with his wife, Beth, and their dog, JoJo. He has two grown children. More information about his books, speaking, private coaching, and schedule can be found at HowardFalco.com and TotalMind-Sports.com and on Instagram and all social media. His foundation to help educate young people on the power of self-awareness, the 8 Wisdom Foundation, can be found at 8Wisdom.org.